AUTOPHAGY

*A Beginner's Guide to Intermittent
Fasting and Metabolic Reset.
Activate the Body's Self-Cleansing
Process to Reduce Inflammation and
Boost Longevity.*

Ashley Brain

Table of Contents

INTRODUCTION

Over the years, living organisms have developed some complex metabolic systems and physiological processes to help them adapt to the environment and its ecological changes.

Daily, we get exposed to infinite numbers of stimuli, that send signals to the body system. This tends to trigger a chain of reactions of evens, which determines how the nervous systems, the metabolism rate, and the psychology will respond.

This book focuses more on autophagy, as a physiological cellular process, which enables the degradation and elimination of the misfolded proteins and the worn out or damaged organelles, which functions in adaptation to cell death, starvation, tumor suppression, and development. This process also entails your healthy living cells, which devours the weak and worn out ones, converting them into energy, this process is literally about your body system eating itself and using it to maintain the process of homeostasis. The cell renewal process that has become associated with nutritional starvation will be discussed extensively in this book.

This book is not about trying to make you live forever; it is an attempt to give to your body the best conditions for longevity and better health performance. It discusses the process of autophagy and its wide belief towards lengthening life span, increasing health performance, and fighting against infectious diseases and cancer.

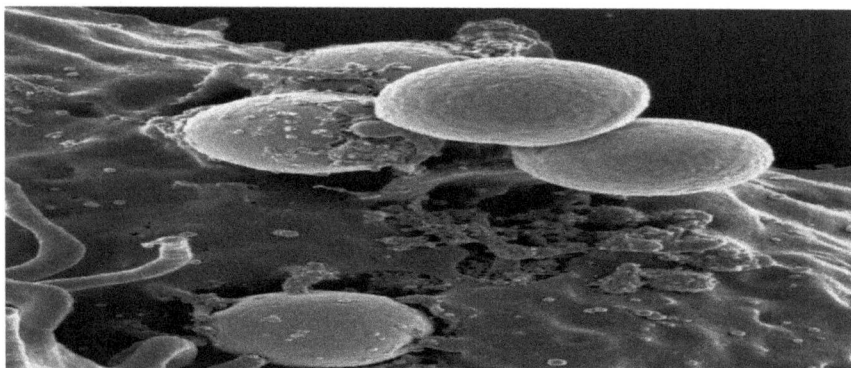

Here is how the book is structured:

➢ In the first chapter, we will be looking deeply into what autophagy is, a detailed explanation of what makes up the process of autophagy, and how it works to enhance the repair and replacement of the worn-out cells and tissues and how it generally helps the body in its miraculous healing mechanism.

Also, in this chapter, we will be giving you an insight into what differentiates the process of autophagy from intermittent fasting. The intermittent fasting will be extensively defined and discussed; a detailed explanation will be made to answer the question of how intermittent fasting triggers the cellular self-healing phenomenon, known as **autophagy.**

➢ The second chapter of this book looks into the types of autophagy. Detailed explanations and analysis will be made on each type of autophagy and each type of autophagy work to fight diseases, through the process of cellular self-digestion. This chapter dishes out to the readers the type of autophagy, classified as either selective or non-selective symbiotic process.

➢ Chapter three of this book introduces and gives a detailed explanation of the benefits of autophagy on a cellular level. It explains deeply, according to some scientific researches and studies, the benefits of autophagy towards enhancing a better skin complexion, a detailed explanation of how it enhances the anti-aging effects, fighting and reduction of the inflammation effects, fight against cancerous cells, and so on.

This chapter also answers the question of how the process of autophagy can be the secret for enhancing life extension.

➤ The fourth chapter of this book introduces to you the tips to activate the process of autophagy in the body system. This chapter will be discussing some of the tools like; dry fasting, intermittent water fasting, exercises,

➤ (the insulin and ketosis). How these tools relate to the process of autophagy and how they all work to activate the process of self-healing phenomenon. We will also be discussing in detail, the five stages of intermittent fasting, and how each stage of intermittent fasting relates to the process of autophagy.

➤ The fifth chapter of this book discusses the type of foods, which promote the process of autophagy. The essential nutrients required during the period of nutritional starvation would be discussed. This chapter also gives a detailed explanation of what type of food to avoid during the period of autophagy. A comprehensive classification of the types of food depending on the available nutrients will be given in this chapter.

The last part of this chapter discusses the time taken for the process of autophagy to kick in.

➤ The sixth chapter of this book discusses the common mistakes made during the process of autophagy; it gives a detailed explanation of the mistakes that could make the process of autophagy stop. Several misconceptions about autophagy are discussed in this chapter, as well as the common myths about the process of autophagy, which has been debunked. All of this will be discussed extensively in this chapter.

➢ The seventh chapter of this book looks into the common healing mistakes which can be encountered during the process of autophagy. All the common mistakes will be listed and adequately discussed; this includes the remedy or steps that can be taken to correct such mistakes made during the nutritional starvation period of autophagy.

This chapter also discusses the common side effects, which are usually associated with autophagy, the causes of these side effects, and the possible steps taken to overcome them.

The effect of detox in autophagy will be discussed extensively in this chapter, an insight on what to expect during this detox period will be discussed, and a detailed explanation on how to deal with the detox.

Some frequently asked questions (FAQS) would also be discussed in full detail. The questions will be answered interactively.

If you think all the details listed above are overwhelming and quite confusing or difficult to understand, I advise you to cast away your worries. From the moment you'll begin to read and devour each page of this book, the vital information in this message will reveal itself to you, and everything will henceforth fall into place for you. Hence, you will be free to make your adjustments based on your lifestyle.

I wish you good luck as you begin your journey towards making the principles and guidelines provided in this book, a permanent part of your life. Be reminded that, for you to be healthier and experience a longer life span, all you have to do is to work daily on the principles discussed in this book.

But before you embark on this journey, let me introduce you to a wise quote, which says;

"The reasonable man adapts himself to the world: the unreasonable one persists in trying to adapt the world to himself. Therefore, all progress depends on the unreasonable man."

George Bernard Shore

CHAPTER ONE
WHAT IS AUTOPHAGY

Autography is derived from the Greek word **"auto"** and **"phage"**; auto means **self** while phage means **eating**. Hence, Autophagy can be defined as a natural, regulated mechanism of the cells, which removes or extracts the unnecessary or dysfunctional components in the body. It is an evolutionarily conserved lysosomal catabolic process, in which the cells of the body degrade and recycle the intracellular endogenous (the worn out or damaged macromolecules, organelles, and mutant proteins) and the exogenous components (such as the viruses and bacteria) to maintain cellular hemostasis.

By removing the damaged part of the cells, autophagy plays a vital role in clearing all the damaged cells structures, such as the mitochondria, endoplasmic reticulum, and the peroxisomes, hence autophagy is often thought of as a survival mechanism.

This catabolic process helps to reduce the aging process, reduces the rate at which dementia is induced, and reduces the risk of cancer. Many cells are required to keep complete functionality for a lifetime; hence, the body knows a unique method for fixing itself and the faulty parts and is able to initiate a defense mechanism that protects itself naturally from all kinds of diseases.

Furthermore, during disease, autophagy has been proven to manifest itself, acting as an adaptive response to stress, hence, promoting the survival of the body cells.

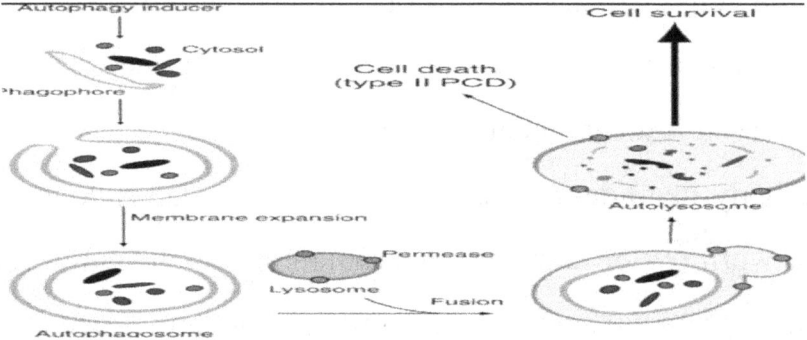

Before we proceed, let's look back into some history:

In the early 1990s, **Yoshinori Ohsumi**, a Japanese Biologist, studied the transport of ions and small molecules in the yeast cell's vacuole, a membrane-bound organelle that corresponds to the lysosome in the human cells. Vacuoles and lysosome act as the waste disposal system of the cell by digesting obsolete material from both inside and outside the cell. Ohsumi reasoned that it could interrupt the degradation process within the vacuole, then autophagy should start and be visible with the aid of a powerful electron microscope.

Ohsumi created mutated yeast cells, which lacked of vacuolar degradation's enzymes and started to starve them. The result was impressive! Within hours, the vacuoles were filled with small vesicles that couldn't be degraded and autophagy started.

Initially, autophagy was thought to be only an hormonal response to starvation or nutritional deficiency, but a recent research has shown that autophagy has several roles in human's physiology too, such as immunity improvement, prevention of genotoxic stress, reduction of inflammation, anti-aging process activation, suppression of cancerous tumor cells and elimination of pathogens.

HOW AUTOPHAGY WORKS TO HELP THE BODY'S MIRACULOUS HEALING MECHANISM

Autophagy is usually activated by nutrient deficiencies and starvation. During t process of nutrient starvation, the insulin goes down, while the glucagon goes up in the body. The increased level of glucagon in the body system stimulates the process of autophagy. In mammalian cells, the complete depletion of amino acids is a very strong signal for autophagy's activation.

During the process of autophagy, the old cell components are broken down into amino acids, which are regarded as the building blocks of proteins. In the early stage of nutrient starvation, the amino acid level will begin to increase. These amino acids are transported straight to the liver for a process known as gluconeogenesis.

There are different types of disorder that the body tries to repair through autophagy:

- **WOUNDS**

During wound healing, injury or pathogenic infection, the skin immune's system will try to halt the ongoing inflammation in order to initiate the restoration process. On these occasions, Rapamycin is released and acts like a powerful autophagy inducer, helping to manage the damage.

- **DIABETES MELLITUS**

People suffering from this disease have insulin deficiencies, conditions that can lead to lesions and ulcers on the skin. In these cases, IRF8, a particular protein produced by the cells induces the Autophagy process, enhancing the chances of self-healing.

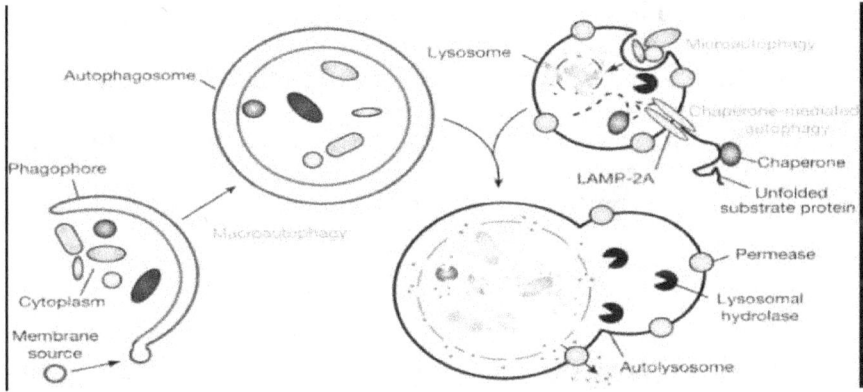

INTERMITTENT FASTING

Intermittent fasting is an eating pattern, that cycles between periods of fasting and eating. Intermittent fasting does not specify WHAT one should eat but, instead, specifies WHEN one should eat. Therefore, it is not considered as a diet in the conventional sense, but it is better described as an eating pattern.

Fasting is a practice, that started a very long time ago, and continued throughout human evolution. The ancient men had no access to refrigerators or food all the time. It could happen that they barely eat for days. The human body then began to develop adaptive behaviors, which enabled itself to function without food for an extended period of time,

However, the science around intermittent fasting is nowadays still preliminary and inconclusive. According to the American Heart Foundation (AHA), intermittent fasting may produce weight loss, reduce insulin resistance, and may have a beneficial cardiometabolic effect, but its long term sustainability is yet to be known.

FASTING AND IMMUNE SYSTEM

The immune system is the most important line of defense against the outside world; it helps fight against foreign intruders that can cause infections, diseases, and other problems.

A fast that lasts from 48 to 120 hours tends to reduce the pro-growth signals responsible for cancer growth and helps to enhance the cellular resistance to toxins. Fasting can also help to stimulate stem cells, reinvigorate old cells and promote the growth of young ones.

In a research study carried out on some chemotherapy patients, who were not fed for several days, it has been seen a significant reduction in the number of white blood cells. This, as a result, turned on the signaling pathways for hematopoietic stem cells (HSC), which are the ones responsible for the generation of blood cells and the immune system.

Therefore, given the evidence of this study, we can say that extended fasting could have a profound impact on the healing rate of your body.

But, how does fasting help in resetting the immune system?

While fasting, the human body starts to mobilize a lot of its internal fuel sources, such as the body fat stores, glycogen, and other cellular debris. Some white blood cells may also be broken down as a result of discarding unnecessary materials.

The intermittent fasting helps to lower the blood sugar, the insulin levels, and other important hormones, such as mTOR and the IGF-1, which are both growth factors that prevent the body from healing itself up by using its internal resources.

INTERMITTENT FASTING AND WEIGHT LOSS

The intermittent fasting is a powerful way of enhancing an effective weight loss. It can decrease the production rate of insulin, fact that leads to a lower rate of nutrient absorption by the cells and may have some beneficial cardiometabolic health effects, although the long term sustainability of all these effects is yet to be proven.

Since the intermittent fasting focuses more on the timing and the frequency of meals than on the type of food you should eat, it's pretty easy to applicate.

Intermittent fasting also helps people to be more conscious about the amount of energy they consume.

HOW THE INTERMITTENT FASTING WORKS

To understand how the intermittent fasting enhances weight or fat loss, we need to understand the difference between the terms; **fed state** and the **fasted state**.

When the body system is in the process of digesting and absorbing food, it is said to be undergoing the fed state. The fed state initiates in the moment that food is being eaten and may last for about two and a half to five hours as the body digests and absorbs the food that has just been eaten. The body hardly burns fat in the fed state, because the insulin level during this period is very high.

After that period, the body transitions itself into another state, which is called the post-absorptive state, which is just a nice way of saying the body is not processing meals. The post-absorptive state may last until approximately 8 to 12 hours after the last meal was eaten, which is when the fasted state was entered. It is much easier for the body to burn fat at this stage because the insulin levels are very low.

In the fasted state, the body becomes capable of burning fats that have been inaccessible during the fed state.

Because the body system does not shift into the fasted state until it is 12 hours after the last meal, it is rare to find the body in the fat-burning state. This is one of the reasons why many people who begin the process of intermittent fasting tend to lose fat without changing the kind of food they eat, the quantity of food they eat, and how frequent they exercise.

Intermittent fasting puts the body in a fat-burning state that one can hardly make it be during a regular eating schedule.

METHODS OF INTERMITTENT FASTING

There are three methods of intermittent fasting; these are:

   i.   Alternate-day fasting

  ii.   Periodic fasting

 iii.   Time-restricted feeding

- **ALTERNATE-DAY FASTING**

The alternate-day fasting involves the alternating between 24 hours when the person consumes less than about 24% of the usual energy needs and a 24-hour non-fasting period. This is the strictest form of intermittent fasting, in the sense that it has more days of fasting in a week.

The alternate-day fasting is further classified into complete alternate-day fasting and the modified alternate-day fasting.

- **COMPLETE ALTERNATE-DAY FASTING**

This is a type of intermittent fasting, in which a person consumes no calories during the period of fasting.

- **MODIFIED ALTERNATE-DAY FASTING**

This type of fasting allows the consumption of about 25 percent of calories daily, during the periods of fasting.

- **PERIODIC FASTING**

This involves a period of fasting, which exceeds 24 hours, such as the five ratios two diets, where there are about one or two fasting days in a week, several days or weeks, in a more extreme version. During the fasting period, about 500 to 600 calories can be taken.

- **TIME RESTRICTED FEEDING**

This type of intermittent fasting involves eating meals during a certain number of hours each day. This schedule is thought to leverage the circadian rhythm.

HEALTHY BENEFITS OF INTERMITTENT FASTING

i. Intermittent fasting may reduce the risk of cancer

Although there is no definitive research and experimental facts or proof on the relationship between fasting and cancer, recent reports seem to be quite positive.

According to the study mentioned before, the side effects of chemotherapy might be drastically reduced by fasting before any treatment is made.

Another study also suggests that people suffering from cancer can have a better cure rate and fewer chances of dying if they fast before undergoing chemotherapy.

Fasting appears not to only to be able to reduce the risk of cancer but also the cardiovascular diseases, by eliminating toxins and promoting the cell viability. This process may also help to fight other diseases like Huntington's and Parkinson's diseases.

A recent study on some women with breast cancer revealed that those who fasted for more than 12 to 13 hours a day had a lower rate of cancer recurrence and progression.

Further researches on intermittent fasting and autophagy are still developing.

ii. Intermittent fasting is capable of increasing one's lifespan

It has long been known by scientific research that restriction of calories is a way of lengthening one's life. From a logical standpoint, this fact makes real sense. When the body is being starved, the body system finds a way of extending its lifespan by eliminating toxins.

Although this may seem quite tricky, it can be mastered with consistent practice. After all, everyone wants to live long. But it comes with a price.

Intermittent fasting tends to activate many of the same mechanisms that are capable of lengthening one's life, the same way as the calorie restriction does.

iii. Intermittent fasting enhances the anti-aging process

By increasing the rate of autophagy, the intermittent fasting stimulates the breakdown and clearance of the damaged or worn-out cell parts. This results in an increased rate of clearance, which is the best way to slow the aging process.

iv. Intermittent fasting is much easier than dieting

One of the reasons why most diet plans fail is because people tend to switch easily to the wrong choice of meal. People do not follow the diet over the long term. It is not a nutrition problem; it is a behavioral problem.

At this instance, intermittent fasting outshines. This is because it is remarkably easy to implement, once the idea that one needs to eat all the time is gotten over. In fact, intermittent fasting is an effective strategy for weight loss, especially in obese adults.

"Diets are easy in the contemplation, difficult in the execution. Intermittent fasting is just the opposite--- it is difficult in the contemplation but easy in the execution.

Most of us have contemplated going on a diet. When we find a diet that appeals to us, it seems as if it will be a breeze to do. But when we get into the nitty-gritty of it, it becomes tough. For example, I stay on a low carb diet almost all the time. But I think about going on a low-fat diet; it looks easy. I think about bagels, whole wheat bread, and jelly, mashed potatoes, corn, bananas by the dozen, etc.—all of which sound appealing. But where am I to embark on such a low-fat diet, I would soon get tired of it and wish I could have meat and eggs? So a diet is easy in contemplation, but not so easy in the long term execution."

Dr. Michael Eades

"Intermittent fasting is hard in the contemplation, of that there is no doubt. "You go without food for 24 hours? People would ask, incredulously when we explain what we are doing. "I could never do that." But once started, it's a snap. No worries about what and where to eat for one or two out of the three meals per day. It is a great liberation.

Your food expenditures plummet. And you are not particularly hungry.

...although it is tough to overcome the idea of doing without food; once you begin the regimen, nothing could be easier."

Dr. Michael Eades

Intermittent fasting is a better option over dieting; it provides a broader range of health benefits without requiring a massive change in lifestyle.

Pitfall prevention!

A popular belief is that intermittent fasting does slow down metabolism in the body... but this is totally wrong!. The intermittent fasting does not slow down the metabolism rate; rather, it increases it by approximately 3.4% after the first 48 hours.

Furthermore, after 4 days, the resting energy expenditure increases up to about 12 to 14%. The body doesn't slow down its metabolism rate, on the contrary! It increases it and pushes it higher. This phenomenon is probably caused by an increase in the level of adrenaline in the system. The scarcer the calories are, the more detrimental, the higher the level of energy and rate of metabolism are.

Usually, people think that if they skip meals, especially breakfast, something negative will happen to their body and they won't be able to get enough energy to live actively...but that's not the truth. The body will sustain itself by utilizing its fat stores.

In the fasted state, the body becomes more efficient with the nutrients gotten from the food we eat, instead of storing up all the food nutrients. With the lack of calories in the body, especially carbohydrates, the body becomes more insulin sensitive, which means that the body needs less insulin to lower the blood sugar levels back to the normal state. Hence, fasting tends to lower the overall blood sugar level by reversing insulin resistance.

It's evident then, that during the intermittent fasting we have no reason to be worried about malnutrition because our body fat stores are capable ok make freeing a big amount of calories.

POTENTIAL SIDE EFFECTS DURING THE INTERMITTENT FASTING

There may also be some possible negative consequences attached to the intermittent fasting. Side effects like headaches, dizziness, fatigue, low blood pressure, and abnormal or irregular heartbeats, all these can occur for a short period of time.

Fasting may lead to the flare-up of certain medical conditions, such as gouts, gallstones, or other diseases. Not all of these conditions are to be considered as a direct result of fasting, but, instead, as a consequence of the overall amount of toxins in the body systems. The adipose tissue in the body is more than a caloric panty; it also stores up infections and poisonous substances that we digest. When the body system starts to breakdown triglycerides, those toxins are re-released into the bloodstreams and need to be flushed out of the body.

Diarrhea may also be experienced, but this can also be considered as a positive effect: fasting is a very effective detox tool, it cleanses the organism entirely and rapidly.

Pitfall prevention!

Fasting is bad for our health.

For a very long time, we have been led to believe that fasting is detrimental to our health. This is wrong!

As arguable or bitter as this sounds, there is no money made from the healthy people who fast!

NOTE:

The intermittent fasting is one of the central cornerstones of the Metabolic Autophagy; this is because it is one of the fewest known ways of activating the process of metabolic autophagy.

WHAT DIFFERENTIATES AUTOPHAGY FROM THE INTERMITTENT FASTING?

The only difference between intermittent fasting and autophagy is that intermittent fasting promotes autophagy. One causes the other.

A high rate of autophagy is typical in young bodies, with the process of aging, the rate of autophagy decreases, and this allows the damaged cells to accumulate. With the help of intermittent fasting, the rate of autophagy can increase again and reach the levels of a younger person.

HOW INTERMITTENT FASTING TRIGGERS AUTOPHAGY

The promotion of autophagy is one of the most significant benefits of intermittent fasting.

While the body is in the fed state, insulin is increased while the rate of autophagy is lowered. During the fasted state, as the level of insulin in the body system drops, the rate of autophagy increases rapidly.

NOTE:

The function of insulin is to promote the increase of the energy storage level and the growth of the organism. The moment the insulin is increased, more fat is stored in the cells, and the other cells use up the glucose from the blood. And most importantly, when the insulin level is increased, the lipids will not be able to leave fat cells. Since to lose fat, we need to get the lipids out of the fat cells in order for them to be burned, we need to put more attention on when/what we eat and how we exercise. These are the key factors to maximize the results.

Actually, intermittent fasting not only stimulates autophagy but is also beneficial for many other functions of the body One of the things that happen during intermittent fasting or starvation is an increase in the rate of amino acid production. The amino acids are delivered to the liver for gluconeogenesis, which is the production of glucose from non-carbohydrate sources (not including fatty-acids). This process leads to the formation of water-soluble molecules called ketone bodies.

Therefore, during the period of fasting, the body system switches from glucose to ketones as a source of energy. This gives a push to the detoxification process at a cellular level.

The reduction of sugar intakes and processed carbs for some hours triggers the mechanism called 'AUTOPHAGY'.

During this process, the body's wastes are recycled into amino acid building blocks that the cells can reuse for repair, while the remaining is eliminated as waste products.

While the body enters the state of ketosis during fasting, the body system tends to undergo a powerful repair mode, which activates or stimulates the higher-order neural networks in the neocortex. This enhances a profound sensation of healing and self-connection.

Even during a short period of starvation, the human growth hormones increase their rate (about 1300 percent), a fact that promotes the process of restoration of the cells that make up the tissues in the body.

While intermittent fasting could be possibly done by everyone, obviously with the due care, long term fasting should not be attempted in patients suffering from diabetes or hypoglycemia until the blood sugar level is regularized.

CHAPTER TWO
TYPES OF AUTOPHAGY

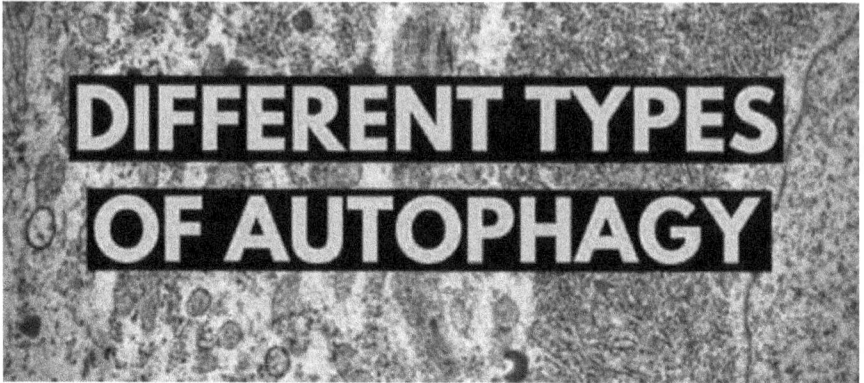

The three main types of autophagy, according to cellular biology, are **Macroautophagy**, **Microautophagy**, and **Chaperone mediated autophagy**.

MICROAUTOPHAGY

Micro autophagy is a term that was first proposed in the year **1966** by **Wattiaux** and **Duve**. It was referred to the hypothetical notion that tiny portions of cytoplasm in the cells of mammals could be directly sequestered and subsequently engulfed by the lysosomes. In contrast with the morphological process of macroautophagy, where the autophagosomes which contain the sequestered cargo subsequently fuses with the lysosomes. In microautophagy, the lysosomal membrane is able to directly engulf the portions of the cytoplasm and any other constituent that need to be absorbed, without the previous activation of autophagosomes. The process of microautophagy involves the direct engulfment of the cytoplasmic material into the lysosomes. This process occurs by invagination, the inward folding of the lysosomal membranes.

The microautophagy's pathways are especially vital for the survival of the cells under the conditions of nutritional starvation, nitrogen deprivation, and after any kind of treatment that involves rapamycin. Although generally, this is a non-selective process, there exist three special cases of selective microautophagy pathways, and they are; micropexophagy, piecemeal microautophagy, and microautophagy. All these are activated under specific conditions.

NON-SELECTIVE MICROAUTOPHAGY

The non-selective microautophagy process can be divided into five distinct steps. The experiments that allowed to observe this process were majorly done on yeasts, nevertheless, the molecular principles seem to be more general and true for human cells as well.

• THE MEMBRANE INVAGINATION

The term invagination can be described as a constitutive process, but its frequency is dramatically increased during periods of nutritional starvation. The membrane invagination is a tubular process, that involves the formation of a structure called "autophagic tube".

The formation of the autophagic tubes is mediated by the activation of the Atg7-dependent ubiquitin or via the vacuolar transporter chaperone (VTC) molecular complex, which tends to act through the calmodulin-dependent manner. The calmodulin involvement in tube formation is a calcium-independent process.

• THE VESICLE FORMATION

The process that stands behind the vesicle formation is based on the lateral sorting mechanism. Changes in the composition of the membrane's molecules (the lipid enrichment in the autophagic tubes is a result of the transmembrane protein removal) lead to the spontaneous formation of the vesicles.

- **THE VESICLE EXPANSION AND SCISSION**

The enlargement of the vesicle is enhanced or stimulated by the binding of the enzymes inside of the unclosed vesicle. The process accompanies the pitch of the vesicle into the lysosomal or vacuolar lumen and is independent from the snare proteins (that are membrane's proteins usually involved in endocytosis).

- **VESICLE DEGRADATION AND RECYCLING**

The vesicle moves freely in the lumen and, after a while, it is degraded by the hydrolases. The Atg22p then releases the nutrients.

THE SELECTIVE MICROAUTOPHAGY

The process of non-selective microautophagy can be observed in all the available types of eukaryotic cells, selective microautophagy, instead, is more commonly observed in yeast cells.

MACROAUTOPHAGY

When we talk about autophagy, we usually refer to macroautophagy. This is a process in which the cells form double-membrane vesicles, called autophagosomes, around a portion of the cytoplasm. The autophagosomes fuse ultimately with the lysosomes, in which their content is released and degraded. Even if usually macroautophagy is stimulated by physiological stress conditions, such as nutritional starvation, is also true that mammalian cells do undergo autophagy at a basal level. This basal activity might be of great importance for the clearance of the frequently occurring, misfolded, and ubiquitylated proteins.

This process is thought to be predominantly a cell-survival mechanism. It is the main pathway used to eradicate or get rid of the dead, damaged (worn-out) cell organelles and used proteins from the body system.

At first, the phagophore engulfs the materials that need to be degraded, envelops it than with a double membrane, known as autophagosome and starts to travel through the cytoplasm of the cell, straight to the lysosomes. Once it gets there, the two organelle fuses. Within the lysosomes, the contents of the autophagosomes are degraded through the action of the acidic lysosomal hydrolases.

Macroautophagy is regulated by the combined activity of autophagy-related and not related genes, which are required for selective sequestration and degradation of some specific cargos.

Macroautophagy plays an essential role in the degradation of a wide range of cellular components, which includes long-lived proteins, protein complexes and aggregates, macromolecules like ribosomes and lipids, organelles such as peroxisomes, endoplasmic reticulum, the nucleus, and mitochondria. The starvation-induced macroautophagy is thought to act in a non-selective manner.

- ## INITIATION OF THE AUTOPHAGOSOMES FORMATION

The autophagosomes formation usually appears to start at the phagophore assembly sites. The source of this membrane is quite unclear, but recent data seems to underline a contribution from the endoplasmic reticulum. The formation of this phagophore requires the activity of the class III phosphoinositide 3-kinase, which forms the phosphoinositide 3-phosphate. The other proteins which are involved in the initiation stages of the formation of the autophagosome are; Atg12, Atg5, Atg16, the newly identified macro autophagy-related protein.

- ## THE AUTOPHAGOSOME ELONGATION

The Atg5 and the Atg12 are widely involved in the first out of the two ubiquitination-like reactions that control the process of macro-autophagy. The Atg12 is conjugated to the Atg5, in a reaction that involves the Atg7 (the ubiquitin-activating enzymes) and the Atg10 (the ubiquitin-conjugating enzyme). The Atg5-Atg12 conjugates are localized onto the PAS and are dissociated upon the completion of the formation of the autophagosomes. The process, which involves the conjugation of the Atg5 and the

Atg12, depends on the Vps34 function, and the Vps34 activity, along with the autophagy, is positively regulated by small GTPase.

The second ubiquitylation-like reaction, involves the conjugation of the microtubule-associated protein one light chain3, to the lipid phosphatidylethanolamine.

- **THE AUTOPHAGOSOMES MATURATION AND FUSION**

The autophagosomes form randomly in the cytoplasm; then, they are moved or transported along the microtubules in a dynein-dependent manner to the lysosomes, which are then clustered around the microtubule-organizing center. The autophagosomes fuse with the lysosomes, and the contents of the two vesicles mix. Enroute to the process of fusion with the lysosomes, the autophagosomes are capable of fusing with the endosomes to form the amphisomes. Although, it is not yet clear whether the amphisome's formation is necessary or even vital for the fusion of the autophagosome-lysosome or not.

THE PHYSIOLOGY AND PATHOLOGY OF MACROAUTOPHAGY

i. NUTRITIONAL STARVATION

One of the long-dated purposes of macroautophagy is to give a push to the process of recycling macromolecules, in order to provide new nutrients if times of starvation occur. This is this type of autophagy's key role in single-cell organisms, such as yeast, and also plays a vital role in mammals as well. For example, in the immediate minutes after a common mice is born, a relative starvation exists before breastfeeding is established. If the mice is autophagy-deficient, modified in the lab, dies sooner, due to its inability to recycle nutrients. Autophagy seems to be pretty vital in these first stages of life.

The macroautophagy can also be essential for the development of mammals as well. Fertilization tends to induce autophagy. Autophagy-defective oocytes, for example, failed in mice to develop beyond the four-cell and eight-cell stages, when fertilized, making it impossible for the embryo to develop.

ii.   AGGREGATION-PRONE PROTEINS

Macro autophagy and the ubiquitin-proteasome system are the key proteolytic systems in mammalian cells. The proteasome can only process the unfolded proteins because it only has a narrow opening: however, the oligomers and the organelles, which are not capable of entering the proteasome, are accessible to autophagy. Macroautophagy plays an essential role in the degradation of the aggregation-prone proteins. These proteins include the neurodegenerative disease-associated proteins, such as the mutant huntingtin, which causes Huntington's disease. Therefore the regulation of autophagy seems to be a possible, powerful, therapeutic strategy for such diseases. Some protein's aggregates that are formed in the brain and some other tissues, contribute to neurogenerative diseases; autophagy could have a key role in the elimination of these complexes.

iii. MACROAUTOPHAGY AND CELL DEATH

Although a considerable number of autophagosomes may sometimes occur in the dying cells, this increase is often not the result of autophagy-mediated cell death.

Autophagy has a cytoprotective role. The process of blocking autophagy tends to increase the susceptibility of cells to proapoptotic insults, whereas, the enhancing autophagy is anti-apoptotic. This is likely because the process of autophagy enhances the clearance of the mitochondria and reduces the mitochondria's load. This allows to diminish the amount of cytochrome c released by the mitochondria that occurs after the apoptotic insult, resulting in less apoptotic's mechanisms activation.

iv. MACRO AUTOPHAGY AND IMMUNITY

Macro autophagy plays a crucial role in the clearance route, for a range of infectious agents, which includes: mycobacterium tuberculosis, streptococcus pyogenes, streptococcal pharyngitis, toxic shock syndrome, the herpes simplex viruses, and the necrotizing fasciitis.

This type of autophagy tends to have positive implications in diseases that are linked to infections, as a route that enables the presentation of cytosolic antigens by the major histocompatibility complex class II molecules, stimulating by doing so an effective defense response.

Studies suggest that autophagy has a wider and important role in thymic epithelial cells, where it regulates the T-cells, and it is crucial for the development of immunological tolerance. This immunological tolerance is accountable for the robust associations of variants in the two autophagy genes.

THE CHAPERONE-MEDIATED AUTOPHAGY (CMA)

The chaperone-mediated autophagy (CMA) is described as the chaperone-dependent selection of the soluble cytosolic proteins, which are then targeted to the lysosomes and directly translocated across the membranes of the lysosomes for the process of degradation to occur.

The most important feature of this type of autophagy is the selectivity made on the proteins, which are degraded by these pathways and the direct shutting of these proteins across the lysosomal membranes, without the requirement for the formation of additional vesicles.

- **THE MOLECULAR COMPONENTS AND THE STEP BY STEP PROCESS OF THE CHAPERONE-MEDIATED AUTOPHAGY (CMA)**

The proteins, that are degraded through the process of chaperone-mediated autophagy, are cytosolic proteins or proteins from other compartments that reach the cytosol stage.

Some of the components that participate in the chaperone-mediated autophagy are present in the cytosol, while others are located in the lysosomal membrane.

Some specific protein's selection mechanisms for the degradation process in all forms of autophagy came to a higher level of understanding as studies discovered the role of the chaperones, like the Hsc70. The Hsc70 works differently, depending on the process it activates, whether the proteins are to be lead to macro or microautophagy, even though it targets the cytosolic protein to the chaperone-mediated autophagy, based on the specific amino acid sequence recognition.

MOLECULAR COMPONENTS OF THE CMA

i. THE SUBSTRATES

This consists of some soluble proteins, such as;

- Aldolase B
- Annexin I
- Annexin II, Annexin III, Annexin IV, and the Annexin VI
- Aspartate aminotransferase, Eps8, and Fos
- Hemoglobin chain, Hsc70, GAPDH
- Pyruvate, Phosphoglycerate mutase
- Kinase, Tau, Ubiquilin, RNase A, RCAN 1, and the substrates of 2OS proteasome.

ROLES/CHARACTERISTICS

- The amount of substrates that undergo the chaperone-mediated autophagy depends on the types and conditions of the cells.
- It recognizes the motif, which is related to the KFERQ.
- The potential substrates are estimated to be an approximate of 30% of cytosolic proteins, according to the linear sequence analysis.

CELLULAR LOCATION

- The cytosol

ii. **CHAPERONES**

This consists of the Cytosolic Hsc70, the lysosome membrane Hsc70, the lysosome lumen Hsc70, the Hsp90.

ROLES/CHARACTERISTICS

- It enhances the substrate's recognition and targeting of the lysosomes.

- It fosters the substrate unfolding, which is assisted by the chaperones.
- It enables the translocations of the substrates.
- It enhances the stability of the receptor's translocation.

CELLULAR LOCATION

- The cytosol

iii. **RECEPTORS**

They consist of the lysosome-associated membrane protein type 2A

ROLES/CHARACTERISTICS

- It enables the process of binding and translocation of the substrates across the membrane by forming a dynamic translocation complex.

CELLULAR LOCATION

- The cytosolic side of the lysosome.

iv. **REGULATORS**

They consist of the EF1 alpha and the GFAP substrates.

ROLES/CHARACTERISTICS

- It increases the multimer stability of the Lamp 2A

- It modulates the association of the GFAP to LAMP-2A

CELLULAR LOCATION

<u>The cytosolic side of the lysosomes.</u>

For a protein to be a CMA substrate, it must have a sequence of pentapeptide motif biochemically, which is related to KFERQ in its amino acid composition. The process of Chaperone-mediated autophagy, targeting motif, is recognized by a cytosolic chaperone, a heat shock cognate protein, that is called 70 kDa (Hsc70), which tends to target the substrate to the surface of the lysosomes.

The substrate protein-chaperone complex that binds to the lysosome-associated membrane protein of type 2A, a single span of protein-membrane, is one of the three spliced variants of the single gene lamp2. The remaining two isoforms, the LAMP2B, and the LAMP2C are usually involved in vesicular trafficking and macroautophagy. The protein substrates do undergo folding after being bound to a LAMP-2A, in a process, which is likely to be mediated by the membrane, associated with the Hsc70 and its co-chaperone. It is also detected in the lysosomal membrane. The process of substrate's translocation requires the presence of the

Hsc70 substrate inside the lysosomal lumen, which may, in turn, act by either pulling the substrates into the lysosomes or preventing their return into the cytosol. After the process of translocation is completed, the substrates proteins are rapidly degraded by the action of the lysosomal proteases.

The only limiting step in the chaperone-mediated autophagy is the process of binding the substrate proteins to the LAMP-2A at the lysosomal membrane, which correlates with the chaperone-mediated autophagy, directly. Hence, to modulate the activity of the autophagic pathway, the cell has to regulate the levels of chaperone-mediated autophagy, stringently at the lysosomal membrane, by controlling the degradation rates of the LAMP-2A monomers in the lysosomes and by de novo synthesis of the LAMP-2A molecules. Also, the transportation of the substrates depends on the efficiency of the assembly of the LAMP-2A into the translocation complex.

Therefore, the assembly and disassembly of the LAMP2-A into the active translocation complex and its degradation in the microdomain regions show the dynamic nature of the process and the importance of the lateral mobility of the chaperone-mediated autophagy (CMA) receptors at the membranes of the lysosomes.

- **PHYSIOLOGICAL FUNCTIONS OF THE CHAPERONE-MEDIATED AUTOPHAGY**

The chaperone-mediated autophagy helps in contributing to the maintenance of the cellular homeostasis by enhancing or stimulating the process of recycling of amino acids of the degraded proteins and elimination of the abnormal or damaged proteins (contribution to the cellular quality control).

The chaperone-mediated autophagy is active at most times in different types of tissues, such as the brain, kidney, and liver, and almost all types of cells in the culture studied. Nevertheless, it is maximally activated in response to the stressors and the changes in their cellular nutritional status.

Whenever the supply of nutrients is limited or insufficient, the cells tend to respond by activating autophagy, to degrade the intracellular components, to provide the energy and building blocks, in which the cells can satisfactory make use of, in the dire state. Normally, autophagy is activated as early as 30 minutes into the period of nutritional starvation, and remains at high activity, for about four to eight hours into the starvation period. But, if the starvation state persists for more than approximately ten hours, the cells tend to switch to the selective formation of the autophagy process, which is called the chaperone-mediated autophagy (CMA), this is known to reach a plateau of a maximal activation of about thirty-five to thirty-six hours into the fasting period maintains these levels for about two to three days.

The chaperone-mediated autophagy is essential in regulating the cellular metabolism process. Specific depletion of the chaperone-mediated autophagy in the liver results in robust hepatic glycogen use, which is accompanied by the accumulation of fat in the liver, along with the altered glucose homeostasis, increased energy expenditures and reduced peripheral adiposity.

The chaperone-mediated autophagy has also been shown by studies to be modulated through the retinoic acid receptor alpha signaling. It is explicitly activated by the designed retinoic and derivatives in the cultured cells.

CMA is responsible for the removal of the damaged and worn out proteins. This function is very critical when the cells are exposed to the agents that cause the protein to be damaged as the selectivity of the CMA ensures that only the damaged or worn-out proteins are targeted to the lysosomes for degradation.

It also performs various specialized functions as well; this depends on the particular proteins which undergo the process of degradation, through this pathway and the type of cells involved. The chaperone-mediated autophagy also contributes to the antigen presentation in the dendritic cells.

NOTE:

The chaperone-mediated autophagy is increased in conjunction with genotoxic stress. Conversely, the decreased chaperone-mediated autophagy activity tends to associate with increased genomes instability and decreased cell survival. The chaperone-mediated autophagy is involved in the removal of the chk1, which is a very important protein for cell cycle progression and the impaired CMA cells.

The chaperone-mediated autophagy also helps to degrade the lipid droplet proteins. The removal of these lipid droplet coat proteins by the CMA precedes the process of lipolysis and lipophagy. This consequently leads the defective chaperone-mediated autophagy activity to massive accumulation of lipid droplets and steatosis.

• PATHOLOGY

The chaperone-mediated autophagy tends to decline with age in many types of cells in humans. This impairment of the CMA in aging is mainly due to a decrease in the levels of the LAMP-2A at the lysosomal membrane. This is because of the reduced stability of the chaperone-mediated receptor and not as a result of the decreased de novo synthesis.

Studies have also shown that there exist links between the chaperone-mediated autophagy (CMA) and cancer. The CMA is usually upregulated in different types of human cancer cells, and the blockage of the CMA in these cells tends to reduce their ability to proliferate, likewise their metastatic and tumorigenic capabilities. In fact, the interference of the LAMP-2A substrate, in the already formed experimental tumors in small mammals, like mice, resulted in their regression.

HOW THE VARIOUS TYPES OF AUTOPHAGY WORK TO FIGHT DISEASES THROUGH CELLULAR SELF DIGESTION

All the types of autophagy, either selective or non-selective, play important roles in human health to help prevent and fight diseases.

The cellular self-digestion can be regarded as a cellular pathway, involved in the degradation of proteins and organelles, with astonishing numbers of connections to human diseases and physiology.

However, the process of autophagy represents a single cell's adaptation to nutritional starvation; if there is a shortage or no available food in the system, the cell would be forced to break down part of its reserves, to stay alive, until this situation improves.

All types of autophagy enhance cytoprotection and cell death. In response to several forms of cellular stress, autophagy plays a cytoprotective role; this is because the

ATG genes-knockdown tends to accelerate cell death, rather than delaying cell death. In the uncontrolled upregulation process of autophagy, this process is capable of enabling the death of cells, through the possible activation of the apoptosis or due to the inability of the cells to survive the non-specific degradation of large amounts of cytoplasmic contents.

In the case of cell deaths in cancer, all the cancerous cells are under the pressure of survival. The failure in apoptosis causes these cells to transform and lead to genetic damage and carcinogenesis. The anti-apoptosis genes are likely to be potential oncogenes, and the cell death genes tend to be a potential tumor suppressor gene.

Furthermore, on starvation, the process of autophagy is heavily increased, this allows the cell to degrade proteins and organelles, and this enables the cell to obtain a source of some macromolecular precursors, such as the amino acids, the fatty acids, and the nucleotides. This makes autophagy play a protective role in enabling the cells to survive during the period of nutrients deprivation.

In addition to the role it plays in cancer death, it is also important in numerous diseases, including bacterial and viral infections, neurodegenerative disorders, cardiovascular diseases, and several myopathies.

CHAPTER THREE

THE BENEFITS OF AUTOPHAGY

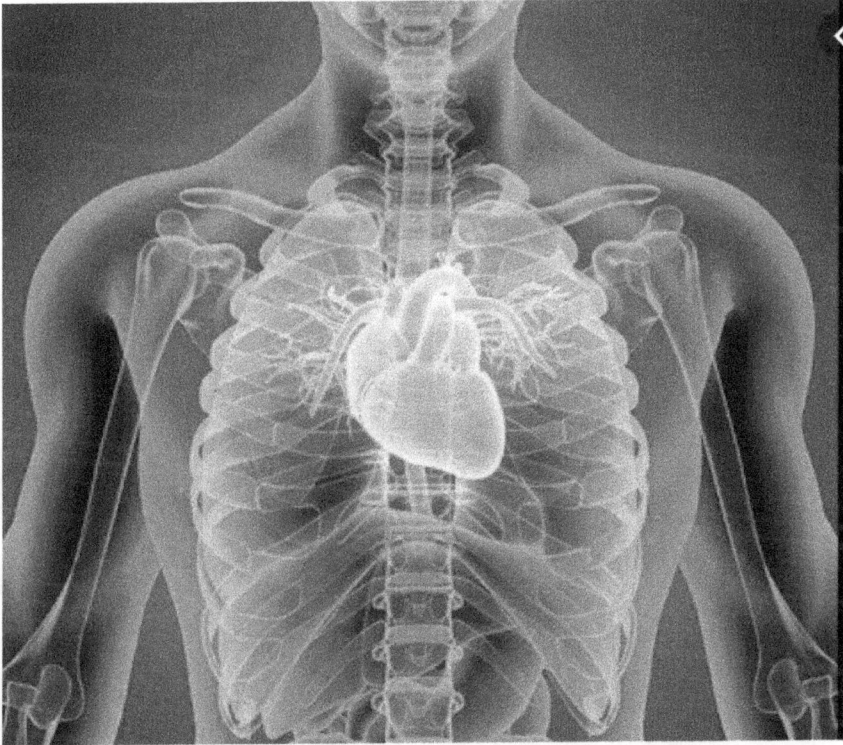

It has been discussed in the previous chapter, that autophagy is an intracellular degradative process, which occurs under stressful conditions; this includes organelle's damage, presence of abnormal proteins and nutritional's deprivation.

Life span and health can be increased or prolonged by the limitation of calories.

Hence, the modulation process of autophagy plays multiple roles in suppressing diseases.

This chapter discusses mainly the benefits of autophagy that can lead to an increased and better lifespan, its actions towards the process of anti-aging and its fight against cancer and inflammation.

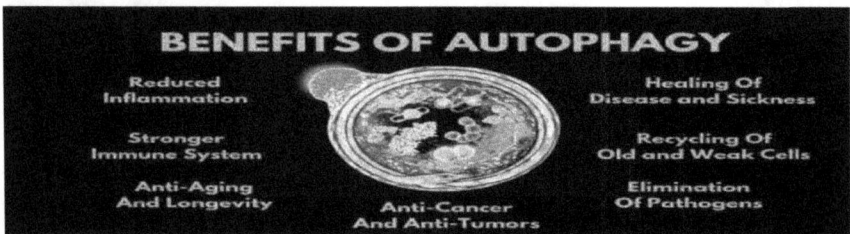

BENEFITS OF AUTOPHAGY

Reduced Inflammation

Healing Of Disease and Sickness

Stronger Immune System

Recycling Of Old and Weak Cells

Anti-Aging And Longevity

Anti-Cancer And Anti-Tumors

Elimination Of Pathogens

Here are listed some of the important autophagy's benefits that can be key points in order to guarantee a better and healthier living:

1. THE ROLE OF AUTOPHAGY IN FIGHTING CANCER

Autophagy plays a vital role in the degradation of the damaged organelles and old proteins, and also in the maintenance of the cellular homeostasis. In the biology of cancer, autophagy plays multiple roles in the suppression of tumors and the development of cancerous cells and proliferation.

Hence, autophagy-regulated chemotherapy can be crucial for the survival or death of the cancerous cells. Furthermore, the process of regulating autophagy contributes towards the expression of the tumor suppressor oncogenes and proteins. The tumor suppressor factors are regulated by the mTOR and the AMPK, thus resulting in the induction of autophagy and suppression of the process that initiates cancer.

- **Autophagy as a regulator of the cancer metastasis**

The cancer cells can engage in metastasis, which is the process of invasion and colonization of the new tissues and the organs via the vascular and lymphatic systems. During the process of metastasis, the cancer cells in the origin experience increased motility to migrate to the secondary sites. In the primary cancer cells, the process of autophagy is induced by the process of nutritional starvation or deprivation, which protects against cell necrosis and inflammation. The process of autophagy is capable of demonstrating an anti-metastatic effect. It does this by limiting the cancer necrosis and response to inflammation in the early stages of the cancer's metastasis.

Autophagy can be considered an anti-metastatic process. The knockdown of the autophagy-related genes, such as the LC3 and the Beclin 1, inhibits proliferation, invasion, and migration, which then leads to apoptosis in breast cancer. A reduction in the ATG5 expression, which is a vital regulator of the autophagy process, reduces the rate of survival in some primary melanoma patients. Studies have shown that blocking mTOR signaling tends to induce autophagic cell death and inhibits metastasis in gastric cancer cells.

The process of autophagy also contributes to the application of immunity in the anticancer therapy process. The immune effects of anticancer therapy occur through some steps. The cancer neoantigens are released into the surrounding environment and are presented to the T cells, which kills the cancerous cells through the T cell-mediated cytotoxicity. The other immune-related cells are also induced and in turn, eliminate the cancer cells presenting the neoantigens through the generation of perforin.

Studies have shown that autophagy may function both as a promoter and a suppressor of the tumor. When used correctly, the modulation of autophagy is a promising potential strategy, which is capable of enhancing cancer therapy. Studies show that the drugs, which target all steps of the autophagic processes from the initiation of the autophagosomes to the process of degradation step, can be crucial. Autophagy, which is enhanced by the process of chemotherapy, can decrease cell death and increases cancer cell survival.

Some of the autophagy's regulators, such as rapamycin, rapamycin water-soluble derivatives, the chloroquine, and the hydroxychloroquine, are used in cancer therapy.

Other autophagy-related drugs have also been developed for anticancer therapy. The spautin-1 inhibits autophagy and leads to the induction of the proteasomal removal of class III PI3K kinase complexes.

- **Autophagy plays a role in preventing cancer onset**

Autophagy is capable of suppressing the cancerous processes, like the chronic inflammation, genome instability, and the DNA damage response. As cancer progresses into malignant stages, it may activate the process of autophagy, to get an alternative fuel. However, the process of autophagy triggers an immune response that affects these cells.

- **THE ROLE OF AUTOPHAGY AS A REGULATOR OF THE TUMOR SUPPRESSION**

Autophagy operates as a mechanism for tumor suppression through the process of reducing the damaged cellular parts, the proteins, and the maintenance of the cellular homeostasis process. Studies have reported that the depletion in the autophagy-related gene, Beclin 1, is observed in a variety of human breasts, prostrates, and ovarian cancers. Beclin 1 is very important in the formation of the phagophore. It is suggested that the Beclin 1 acts as a tumor suppressor. In an experiment made on mice, the loss of the gene BECN1 resulted in the reduction of the autophagy process and an increase in cell proliferation; this further indicated that the BECN1 gene acts as a tumor suppressor. Studies have also shown or revealed that the level of beclin 1 is decreased in several cancer cells, such as cervical squamous-cell carcinomas and hepatocellular carcinomas. Hence, the process of autophagy prevents the generation of tumors through the process of regulating reactive oxygen species (ROS). The damage done to the mitochondria induces the excessive production of the reactive oxygen species, thus leading to the promotion of the carcinogenesis process. This suggests that the process of autophagy is a crucial mechanism, which enhances the tumor generation, and the impaired autophagy may lead to the occurrence of oncogenesis.

- ## THE ROLE OF AUTOPHAGY IN CANCER STEM CELLS

The cancer stem cells are a tiny population of the cancerous cells, which have the ability of self-renewal and to differentiate themselves.; abilities that contribute to the tumor initiation process, the chemoresistance, and the metastasis process. Studies have investigated the role of autophagy in the maintenance of the stemness process. These studies have shown that the process of autophagy promotes differentiation. The decrease in the quantity of the Beclin-1 and the LC3B-II are related to the development of the astrocytic tumors. However, one of the studies revealed that autophagic cell death is observed in the glioma cells, but it's still unclear whether autophagy regulates the stemness in the glioma stem cells or not.

In the breast cancer's stem cells, studies revealed that the CSCs played a vital role in the recurrence of cancer and metastasis process. The process of autophagy has been observed to modulate the Mesenchymal-like Phenotypes in the breast cancer's stem cells, in a positive manner. The process of silencing the two autophagy-related proteins, ATG12, and the LC3B or the treatment, with the autophagy inhibitors, directly reduces the cancer stem-cell-like phenotypes. Studies have repeatedly shown that autophagy is associated or related to the protective effects against the various cellular stress in breast CSCs.

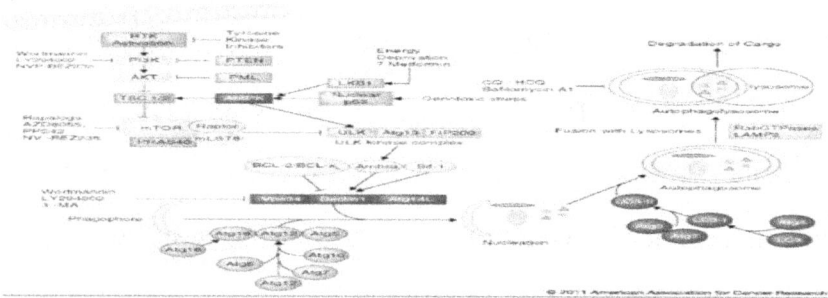

© 2011 American Association for Cancer Research

2. THE ROLE OF AUTOPHAGY TOWARDS ANTI-AGING

The process of autophagy and aging seem to be interwoven or connected. When the genes that stimulate autophagy are inhibited in the mammalian cells, degeneration is said to occur. Whenever autophagy is enhanced during some lifespan-extending therapies, such as the insulin growth factor pathway inhibition, the calorie restriction, rapamycin, resveratrol, and the spermidine, the anti-aging effects seem to be suppressed.

Autophagy has some benefits in the study of age-related diseases, such as atherosclerosis. Atherosclerosis is said to be a circulatory disease characterized by the hardening and narrowing of the arteries, which is caused by the formation of plaques. Hence, atherosclerosis can furtherly lead to strokes, heart attacks, and other circulatory diseases.

Studies established that there is a connection between a reduced autophagy and the formation of the plaques, which are responsible for atherosclerosis. Scientists, who bred mice for experimental purposes, explained that the mice enhanced autophagy by increasing the expression of the gene called the TFEB. The change that occurred seemed to have some protective effects against atherosclerosis, which was caused by a western diet. Also, they further showed that trehalose, a naturally occurring sugar, enhances the process of autophagy. This reduced the signs of atherosclerosis when it was injected into the body cavities of the mice.

Even if the antiaging benefits of autophagy may sound too good to be true, they are. Instead of the cells to take a new nutrient, the cells, which are, undergoing the process of autophagy, recycle the damaged parts that they have, thereby removing the toxic material. When the cells repair themselves, they tend to work better, and they, as a result, behave like younger cells.

3. THE ROLE OF AUTOPHAGY IN FIGHTING AND REDUCING INFLAMMATION

There is a complex association between autophagy and inflammation. Autophagy influences the development, homeostasis, and survival of the inflammatory cells, which include the macrophages, the neutrophils, and the lymphocytes, which play vital roles in the development and the process of the pathogenesis of inflammation.

The macrophages are essential or vital for the host's defense system. As a type of phagocytes, they are capable of uptaking and kill the pathogens intracellularly, as well as producing the inflammatory cytokines and the chemokines. Studies have shown that autophagy contributed to the execution of the caspase-independent cell death in activated macrophages. This study detected an increase in the poly polymerase activation and the reactive oxygen species production in the lipopolysaccharide-treated macrophages, accompanied by the formation of the autophagic bodies and the macrophage cell's death. The death of these activated macrophages could be beneficial in controlling the level of inflammation.

The neutrophils are multifunctional; these cells play a central role in the innate immune system. The inflammatory stimuli attract the neutrophils to the infected tissues, where they engulf and inactivate the microorganisms through the fusion of the phagosomes, with granules and the formation of phagolysosomes, in which the antimicrobial peptides and the ROS tends to act synergistically for the clearance of the pathogens. The neutrophil's apoptosis contributes to the resolution of inflammation.

Studies have shown that autophagy plays an essential role in both acute and chronic inflammatory processes. Thereby, it can potentially have an essential impact on the outcome of the disease's progression.

For instance, in the case of Mycobacterium tuberculosis, an intracellular pathogen that persists within the phagosomes through the interference with the phagolysosomes biogenesis, the experimental simulation of the process of autophagy is capable of overcoming the trafficking block imposed by the bacteria.

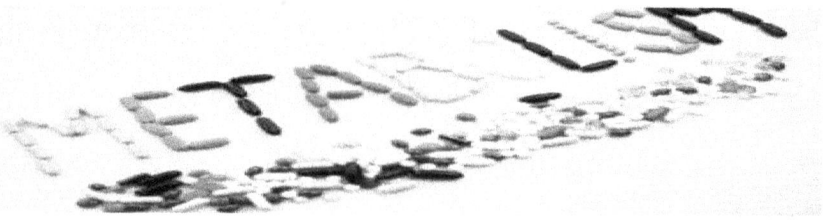

NOTE:

We have discussed the role of the process of autophagy in the pathogenesis of inflammation, including the elimination of the pathogens, the regulation of innate and adaptive immune response. We also discussed the potential therapeutic role of autophagy in inflammatory diseases. Recent shreds of evidence have also shown or identified its roles in the process of carcinogenesis. This implicates that autophagy is an important or essential modulator of disease's pathogenesis. The bacterial clearing function of autophagy may likely contribute to hosts of defenses in the diseases involving bacteria, such as the inflammatory disease, strepsils, and respiratory infections. The process of autophagy may also play a vital role in the downregulating pro-inflammatory diseases, which does not necessarily involve bacterial infection. Although some significant progress has been made in the role of autophagy in inflammation, it has to be understood that the knowledge on molecular's mechanism and pathways of autophagy and its relationship with the inflammatory diseases, is still quite primitive, for now.

4. THE ROLE OF AUTOPHAGY IN METABOLISM

Autophagy is the process of taking out damaged or worn-out cells and replacing them with new cell parts like the Mitochondria. The mitochondria are the cellular engines of the body system. They help to burn the fats in the body systems and convert them to ATP, the body's energetic currency. There are numerous toxic components that are created in the mitochondria, that are capable of causing damages to the cells. Breaking them down saves the cells from self-degradation and toxicity in the future. The autophagy of the other cell's parts helps not only to burn the fuel, but also works more efficiently, not to burn the fuel only, but to produce or make proteins.

5. THE ROLE OF AUTOPHAGY IN THE REDUCTION OF NEURODEGENERATIVE DISEASES

Numerous diseases, which involve the aging of the brain, take a long time to develop because they are the result of some altered proteins that slowly accumulate in and around the brain cells. The process of autophagy helps the cells to clean up the proteins that are not performing their functions properly, preventing the body to accumulate them. For example, Alzheimer's disease autophagy removes the amyloid, a protein complex involved in the appearance of the illness, while in Parkinson's disease autophagy removes the alpha-synuclein.

6. THE ROLE OF AUTOPHAGY IN THE LIFE SPAN EXTENSION

This is one of the main benefits of autophagy; it breaks down the damaged organelles, proteins, RNA sequences, and cell membranes. All these eventually build up the body system over time. The proteins and the majority of the organelle can repair themselves whenever they are damaged. These worn out and damaged cells become a drain on the body's resources at its best, and a potential source of cancer, in the worst condition.

The most significant fact is that the death of the cell is vital or very important for the extension of lifespan and limitation of the aging effect.

Studies have shown that the process of autophagy improves cellular's health in the body system. Instead of producing or taking in fresh nutrients, the cells, which undergoes autophagy, tend to repair the damaged parts that they have, removing all the toxic or harmful materials in the system, behaving then, like the younger cells again.

7. AUTOPHAGY IMPROVES THE MUSCULAR PERFORMANCE

When micro-tears and inflammation appear during exercise, the muscles need to be repaired and the demand for energy needed will be increased. The muscles cells will respond to this request by activating the process of autophagy. This will reduce the energy's demands of the muscles, thanks to the degradation of the damaged components, and hence, will improve then the general energy's balance in the body system. Furthermore, thanks to this autophagy's activation, risks of future damages will be reduced.

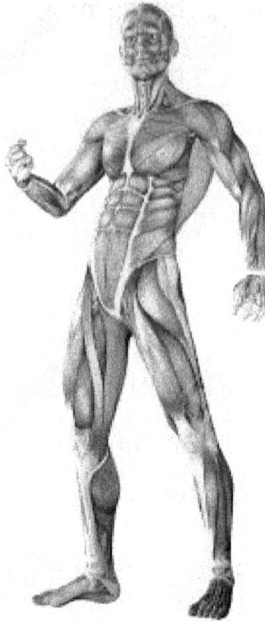

8. THE ROLE OF AUTOPHAGY, IN IMPROVING THE DIGESTIVE HEALTH

The cells that cover the gastrointestinal tracts are always required to do some kind of work. They work so hard that they need to be often renewed and replaced, the old ones are constantly expelled through the feces. Autophagy plays an important role in this renewal and reparation's process, it allows, in fact, to restore the old cells and eliminate the damaged ones. This process is capable of increasing and reducing the immune system. Be aware that in case of the presence of chronic immune response in the gut, capable of overwhelming and inflaming the bowels, the gut will require some time to repair, rest, and restore its self.

9. AUTOPHAGY PLAYS A ROLE IN ENHANCING AN HEALTHY WEIGHT

In its early phases, the process of autophagy involves mostly the fat-burning paths and tends to not utilize the protein's ones. It's only after a prolonged nutritional starvation that there will be a loss in the protein mass. That's why shorter periods of nutritional starvation are better: autophagy will be activated but only fats will be burned, this is the best wat to get a healthier and fitter you.

10. AUTOPHAGY MINIMIZES THE APOPTOSIS PROCESS (THE PROGRAMMED DEATH OF A CELL)

Apoptosis can be defined as the death of a cell. The dead cell becomes a product of waste for the body system, in fact, the body needs to replace and get rid of it. To do so, the body system triggers the process of inflammation and cleans up the dead cells. The more the number of cells, which repair themselves before they get damaged or worn out, the lesser the efforts required by the body system to clean up and replace these cells. Thanks to the work done by Autophagy, during tissue renewal less inflammation will be required.

11. THE ROLE OF AUTOPHAGY TOWARDS IMPROVING THE SKIN COMPLEXION

The collagen and the basic skin's functions tend to deteriorate as we become older. Autophagy is one of the tools that can help save the skin complexion.

The collagen and the elastin of the skin, which are located in the dermis layer, tend to deteriorate at a ratio of about one percent every year. When the process of autophagy is activated, it's not only able to improve the amount of collagen and elastin cells, that are present in the skin but also to make them act like they did when they were younger.

Hence, thanks to autophagy, the body system will be able again to restore its cell cycle, by speeding up the cell turnover; the body will tend to boost the collagen out more efficiently and this will give a more youthful glow.

12. THE ROLE OF AUTOPHAGY IN PHYSICAL FITNESS

The process of autophagy plays an important role both during exercise and post exercise's recovery.

During physical exercise, the process of macroautophagy is required to maintain the glucose homeostasis and the amino acid reserved within the cells of the muscles. Without the process of autophagy, the cells would quickly run out of energy during physical effort, especially during aerobic exercises. Without autophagy, exercises could become detrimental for the health; after all, what physical activity initially does is to damage the body; the body system only fights back and becomes stronger after fully recovering from the damage.

Exercise leads to muscular degeneration; this is the consequence of the buildup of the damaged mitochondria, located inside of the muscle cells. This dramatically leads to an increase in the rate of death among the muscle cells. The introduction of autophagy is able to reverse the damages.

It's also important to say that the process of autophagy contributes to many other benefits that accompany exercises, it improves the body's stamina, the muscle's mass, and the bone's mass as well.

In conclusion, when you grow older, the process of autophagy is an important angle to be considered if you want to stay healthy, especially if you want to enhance your athletic performances.

Pitfall prevention!

There is a wide belief that the process of autophagy may help reduce or eat up wrinkles and support a loose skin, this is a misconception because the process does not literally eat up the wrinkles, it only supports the processes that allows the skin to be more elastic and able to tighten up faster.

However, in the case of an extreme weight loss, the process of fasting and autophagy can help prevent excessive loose skin. After some weight is lost, loose skin can be present, but if the weight is lost through the process of nutritional starvation, there will be enough autophagy to help the skin adapt to the new weight quickly.

Diets with restricted calorie intake and autophagy are more likely to create loose skin; this is due to the fact that autophagy has a central role in keeping the fibroblasts and the production of collagen very active.

Loose skin usually occur because the skin is a massive portion of tissues, that expands and contracts when it is required, that's why the elastic layers stretch out as the body gains weight. Loose skins could also occur when the skin is not healthy enough to possess the elasticity property.

Consider that, when there is a loss of fat in the body system, thanks to autophagy, the skin will naturally tighten itself up. This is because there will be less mass underneath.

IS AUTOPHAGY THE SECRETE TO LIFE EXTENSION?

The study of human longevity and lifespan extension is quite difficult; this is because scientists cannot spend years manipulating someone's autophagic processes to determine if it makes them live for a longer time or die sooner. However, this can be done in animals. Studies have shown that, on the whole, animal models tend to live longer when the process of autophagy is upregulated, and die younger or sooner when it is prevented.

Our basic knowledge of autophagy centers on the recycling of the damaged cell components, such as the cytoplasm, the organelles, and the proteins, which helps the cells to live for a longer period. The entire cell may sometimes become irreparably damaged, this can be caused by stressors like infections and radiations or because the cell has become too old or has been already replicated a lot of times. This phenomenon is called **cellular senescence**.

Hence, it's important to say that programmed cell death, like autophagy, is responsible for extending lifespan and limiting the effects of the aging process.

Autophagy is, therefore, a secret for extending lifespan, but it is possible that in some circumstances, the process of autophagy may work against one of the anti-aging mechanisms of the human body, but more research is required in this area.

CHAPTER FOUR
TIPS TO ACTIVATE AUTOPHAGY

The process of autophagy can be practiced; the body can be trained to eat itself up. This is a natural process, and it is the system that the body uses for cleaning the house. The cells in the body create membranes that usually hunt or scout out the damaged, dead, or worn-out cells or tissues, the system just have to recognize them. Once these waste products are degraded, the body uses the resulting molecules to create energy or make new types of cell parts.

Firstly, autophagy can be said to be a response to stress; the body will have to undergo some stress in order to stimulate a little extra auto cannibalism. Hence, a short-term discomfort (like a brief fast) can bring a long-term benefit.

This chapter discusses the tips to activate the process of autophagy. We will talk about the tools that will help you to initiate the process.

Here are some of the best ways to activate the process of autophagy:

1. INTERMITTENT FASTING

Intermittent fasting refers to a process of abstaining from food or particular essential nutrients at a specific time. It consists of two integral parts, the fasting time and the eating time. The body is wholly deprived of all types of food or nutrients that may provide a certain amount of calories during the fasting period. There is, however, another type of fasting or nutritional deprivation that embraces or requires water to be consumed. This is called intermittent water fasting.

Intermittent fasting is not a magical activity that triggers the process of excessive weight loss. Nonetheless, it is a mechanism that can activate the cycle of autophagy and should be perceived as a tool that can be used to improve health. Studies have shown that intermittent fasting is an option for balanced and healthy weight loss and calorie intake control.

NOTE:

The process of intermittent fasting is the most significant and proven way to trigger the process of autophagy. The signaling of autophagy in the body involves the two most essential pathways that occur when the body becomes nutritionally deprived.

The mTOR (mammalian target of rapamycin) regulates the nutrients that affect the cellular growth, the anabolic process and the synthesis process in the body system. This process is usually linked to the activation of the insulin receptors and the creation of new tissues.

The AMP-activated protein kinase helps the body to maintain the energy homeostasis and hence, activates the backup fuel mechanisms of the body.

Despite the excellent benefits that accompany this process, you have to consider that the required level of fasting, which will activate or trigger autophagy, is not the same for everybody.

How does the intermittent fasting work?

To understand how intermittent fasting activates the process of autophagy, we need to understand the difference between these two terms; **the fed state** and **the fasted state**.

The body is said to be in the fed state when it is undergoing the process of nutrient digestion and absorption. The fed state begins when you start to eat, and it lasts for about five hours as the body digests and absorbs all the nutrients from the meal you've just eaten. When you are in the fed state your body doesn't burn stored fats because the insulin levels are very high and promote accumulation rather than degradation. After this period, the body goes into the post-absorptive state, which lasts for about seven to thirteen hours after the last meal was eaten, only after this phase the body enters the fasted state.

During the fasted state, the body system becomes capable of burning fats, which were inaccessible during the fed state.

DRY INTERMITTENT FASTING AND WATER INTERMITTENT FASTING

- **DRY FASTING**

It's the advanced version of the intermittent fasting, where it is not only the calories that are being avoided but also the consumption of water and other types of liquids.

During the period of dry fasting, the body system begins to get its water from the cells. Approximately, about 60% of the body is made of H_2O molecules, this is the main component of the cells and, therefore, of the organs and the muscles as well. Cell's dehydration inhibits the mTOR signaling and raises the AMPK; as a result, we'll notice an important increase in the rate at which autophagy occurs.

Therefore, since it allows stress levels to exponentially grow, dry fasting is capable of a powerful activation of autophagy.

- **WATER FASTING**

Water fasting is a period of fasting in which the body is completely deprived of food and every other liquid, except for water. This type of fasting is vital for weight loss and it is very safe at the same time. Furthermore, this method of fasting, when made correctly and consciously, could lead to a reduction in the appearance of cancer and diabetes.

Pitfall prevention!

When considering intermittent fasting, you should discuss it with your doctor. Skipping meals and limiting the intake of calories can be dangerous for people with certain medical conditions, such as diabetes, heart diseases, unstable blood pressures. People with such medical conditions may render themselves prone to some abnormalities in their body electrolyte's balance.

BENEFITS OF THE INTERMITTENT FASTING

- **It extends the life-span of an individual**

The intermittent fasting, thanks to the calorie restriction that it gives, helps to activate the various mechanisms that are responsible for extending the lifespan. There are many studies that have been trying to understand the link or connection between intermittent fasting and longevity.

The findings of these research reveal that restricting calorie intake tends to turn on the genes that instruct the cells to preserve their resources. These cells tend to go into a state known as the famine mode. This phase allows them to be are remarkably more resistant to diseases or cellular stress. The cells also enter the process of autophagy, where the body system begins to wipe out the damaged, worn out and unwanted cellular materials, as well as fixing and recycling the damaged cell parts. The process of autophagy is initiated in humans after about 18 to 20 hours of fasting, while the maximum effect of the process can be seen after about 48 hours of food's absence.

The process of autophagy allows a lot of positive things to happen: it wipes out the damaged, worn out and unwanted cells and proteins and it enhances the production of the growth hormones, which tend to regenerate fresh cellular materials. The process of autophagy is not only linked to an increased lifespan, but also to the fight against degenerative diseases.

- **It enhances Carb Cycling**

Carb cycling can be described as a dietary approach, in which one alternates the intake of carbs on a daily, weekly, or monthly basis.

This process enhances autophagy in the sense that it helps to limit the intake of carbs. Carb cycling is commonly used to lose fat and to maintain a physical performance while dieting. This process aims to limit the carbohydrate intake when it provides the maximum benefit and excludes the carbs when they are not required.

Many people will cycle their intake of carbohydrates based on the level of body fat they have. The leaner they become, the more days of high-carb they include.

Hence, by having scheduled periods of high-carb and low-carbs meals, one may enjoy the numerous benefits provided by both diets, without experiencing the negative side effects. The low-carb period aids better insulin sensitivity, increased burning of fats, enhanced metabolic health, and an improved level of cholesterol in the body while the high-carb provides some positive effects on the hormones, like the thyroid hormones, the leptin, and the testosterone.

2. KETOSIS

Even if fasting, as a way to induce the process of autophagy, has numerous benefits beyond activating autophagy, it may not always be possible. In these cases, ketosis is capable of delivering the same benefits.

WHAT IS KETOSIS?

This is a state in which the body makes use of the fats, instead of the glucose, as a source of energy. Ketosis can be achieved without eliminating food or undergoing the process of nutritional starvation. You will be instructed to eat highly fatty food, moderate protein, and a low carb diet, just like the ketogenic diet.

This type of diet tends to reduce the carb content so that the body is forced to start utilizing the fat in order to obtain fuel. The process of practicing ketosis is capable of having a huge impact on cellular health.

Hence, to activate the process of autophagy from ketosis, you have to make sure that you are not eating too much in the usual manner. You will be practicing some form of time-restricted eating, you won't eat too many carbs and proteins and you will give more space to physical activity.

Many people think that the ketogenic diet is the best way to trigger the process of autophagy and to reduce the consumption of protein. This is important because proteins can turn into sugar when you consume too much of them.

To fats, this doesn't happen. When high fat, low protein, and low carb diets are consumed, the body shifts the fuel's source to ketones, a fact that tends to mimic the effects of the fasted state.

This process reduces the toxins in the body, leaving less work to autophagy.

HOW TO TEST FOR KETOSIS

The keto Mojo meter can be used to determine if you are in the state of ketosis or not. This meter measures a small drop of blood and tests the level of the blood's ketone. A standard nutritional ketosis is considered to be at the level of about 0.5mmol/L to 1.5mmol/L, while 1.5mmol/L to 3mmol/L is considered optimal in order to activate the fat burning process and, potentially, autophagy.

BENEFITS OF KETOSIS

The ketogenic diet has been proposed as a potential adjuvant therapy during cancer. It's able to exploit, in fact, the differences between the cancerogenic and the normal cells. The consumption of a ketogenic diet tends to reduce the level of glucose in the blood, through a drastic reduction or decrement in the number of carbs consumed. Thanks to a decrease in the level of blood's glucose, less amount of insulin is secreted, a fact that tends to downregulate the signaling pathways that are frequently active in the tumor cells. Glucose metabolism is inhibited and energy must be primarily derived from the fats. The fat metabolism then results in the production of ketone bodies and beta-hydroxybutyrate by the liver; which is used for the production of fuel energy. Luckily, It is quite difficult for the cancer cells to make use of these pathways because they primarily rely on glucose.

Protein metabolism too forces the cells to make use of the amino acids, rather than the glucose, to produce energy, nevertheless, studies have suggested that it does not cause the same level of oxidative stress that the metabolism of fat does.

Furthermore, the overall success of the ketogenic diet in animals has increased the interest of adopting this diet in patients' diets as well.

Lastly, studies suggest that the ketogenic diet may be an effective adjunct towards cancer treatment, although some cancer such as those in the kidney may not benefit. Non-human-based researches have found that the ketogenic diet could be harmful or toxic for these patients.

3. EXERCISES

Exercising improves health in the long term through the mechanism of increased autophagy and the collection of cellular maintenance processes, which are activated by various stressors. The lack of nutrients, combined with the oxidative molecules that are generated during the hard physical work, are sufficient to trigger or activate a higher level of autophagy, that continues after the stress has ended.

Studies have found that daily exercises help to sensitize the autophagic system, which facilitates the elimination of the proteins and the organelles, which are not functional in the muscles. The removal of these dysfunctional components is very vital or essential; this is because, when they accumulate, they become toxic and then contribute to the impairment of the muscle cell, leading to cell death. If we imagine the muscles as a refrigerator, the neurons from which they are innervated are the electric cables that give the energy needed. If the signal is suddenly interrupted because the plug is forcefully pulled out of the power source, the food in the fridge, and so the proteins in the muscles, would start to spoil at different speed rates, according to their various compositions. At this point, an early warning mechanism, which is present in the cells but not in the fridge, tends to activate the autophagic system, which isolates, identifies, and incinerates the defective material; this prevents the propagation of the damage. If the muscles do not receive the right electric signal for a long time, the early warning mechanism tends to stop working efficiently and the cells slowly start to collapse.

During an intense and acute physical exercise, the energy's stores of the targeted muscle tissues are fully utilized, this process induces autophagy. Autophagy plays an essential role in maintaining cellular energy stores during exercise. About 60 minutes of exercise, done at a moderate speed, are enough to trigger or activate autophagy. The physical activity does not only trigger autophagy in that specific moment, but it also increases the body's general capacity to activate autophagy every time it needs to adapt to exercises. Studies revealed that the process of autophagy is more readily induced when exercise becomes more intense, the study also noted that autophagy occurs more readily when the physical activity is done during the fasted state. This is quite obvious since autophagy is induced during moments of lack of nutritional resources.

The study also revealed that muscle's autophagy begins to be less intense after about 1 to 2 hours of moderate-intensity exercise or about 20 minutes of low-intensity exercise.

NOTE:

Unlike fasting and ketosis, exercise tends to deplete the energy that is reserved in the specific muscle's cells that were involved in the exercise and not the whole body. Autophagy activates then just in these specific areas, at least until you exercise for a greater period of time, which is long enough to cause a depletion in the glycogen level in the entire body. Hence, the exercise-induced autophagy should be considered as a way to improve athletic performances, while the diet-induced autophagy's process is more useful to obtain life extension and cancer prevention.

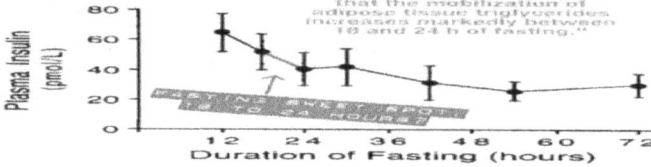

"Of the total increase in lipid kinetics, 60% occurred between 12 and 24 h of fasting; the greatest interval change occured between 18 and 24 h of fasting."

"Plasma insulin decreased by ~50% between 12 h and 72 h of fasting. Of the total decline in plasma insulin, 70% occurred within the first 24 h of fasting."

"These results demonstrate that the mobilization of adipose tissue triglycerides increases markedly between 18 and 24 h of fasting."

HOW THE FIVE STAGES OF INTERMITTENT FASTING RELATE TO AUTOPHAGY

- **By 12 hours of fasting, you should enter the metabolic state, which is called ketosis.**

  Some of the fat, that is used by the liver to produce the ketone bodies, serves as an alternative source of energy for the cells that are in the tissues where glucose is not available. During fasting, the ketone bodies, which are generated by the liver, partly replace the glucose as fuel for the brain and other organs in the body. The ketones usage by the brain is one of the main reasons why fasting is often claimed to promote the process of mental clarity and positive mood. The ketones produce less inflammatory products than the glucose, and they are capable of kick-starting the production of the brain's growth factor.

- **By 18 hours should have switched to the fat-burning mode; this enables to generate a more significant quantity of ketones**

At this point, the ketone's levels in the blood are above the baseline values of about 0.6 to 1.0.

As the level of ketones in the bloodstream rises or increases, the ketones tend to act as signaling molecules, that are similar to hormones and start to tell the body to ramp up the stress-busting pathways that reduce the inflammation and repair the damaged DNA.

- **Within 24 hours, the cells in the body increasingly recycle the old components and break down the misfolded proteins that are linked to infectious diseases (we are now in the already well-known process called autophagy).**

When the cells in the body cannot or do not initiate the process of autophagy, non-positive things start to happen, like neurodegenerative diseases. The process of autophagy is significant for cells and tissue rejuvenation. This process removes the damaged cellular components, like the dangerous misfolded protein. Fasting tends to activate the AMPK signaling pathway and then inhibits the mTOR activity, a fact that also contributes to the activation of autophagy. This process starts only when the body depletes the glucose stores, which results in a drop in the insulin level.

- **By 48 hours, the body experiences a peak in the levels of the growth hormone. In fact, after 2 days spent without any or with a minimal amount of calories intake (no proteins, no carbs), the body's growth hormone's level becomes five times as high as when you first started to fast.**

One of the causes of this increase is that the ketone bodies, which are produced during the period of fasting, tend to promote the secretion of this hormone. The growth hormones tend to help in preserving the lean muscle mass and reduces fatty tissue accumulation, especially as we get older. It also plays a role in the expansion's process of lifespan in mammals and promotes the healing of wounds and cardiovascular health.

- **By 54 hours, the body experiences a minimum in the insulin's production, its level drops to its lowest since the fasting process was started.**

Lowering the insulin level has a range of health benefits, both for the short and long term. A lowered level of insulin, puts a brake on the insulin and mTOR signaling pathways, thus activating autophagy. The lowered insulin level can reduce inflammation and make the body more sensitive and hence, protect the body from the chronic diseases connected with the process of aging, including cancer.

- **By 72 hours, the body breaks down the old immune cells and generates new ones.**

Prolonged fasting will reduce the circulation of the IGF-1, the insulin-like growth factor 1, which is similar to the insulin and has growth-promoting effects. The IGF-1 activates the signaling pathways, which include the PI3K-Akt pathway that promotes cell growth and survival mechanisms. The PKA is also capable of activating the mTOR pathway. This process can turn down the cellular survival pathways and lead to the breakdown and recycling of the old cells and proteins. The prolonged fasting (about 72 hours) has been proven to be able to help in the preservation of the healthy white blood cells and lymphocytes in the body of the patients who are undergoing chemotherapy.

CHAPTER FIVE

FOODS THAT PROMOTE AUTOPHAGY

"It always seems impossible until it is done"

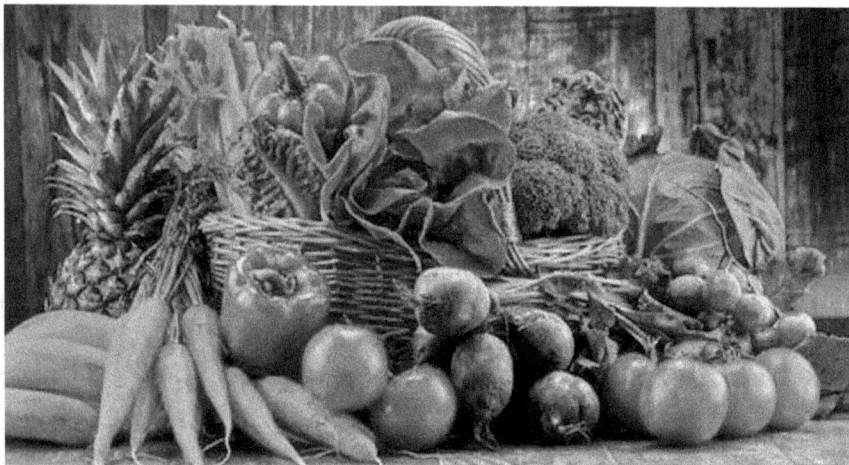

As discussed in the previous chapters, autophagy is an important mechanism of self-healing in the body system. The process of autophagy can be triggered when the body is being subjected to nutritional starvation.

The practice of autophagy does not necessarily require the complete deprivation of the required nutrients. There are some nutrients, whether macro or micro, that help to boost this metabolic process. Nutrients like proteins, low-carb meals, animal fat, potassium, calcium, phosphorus are important for the body to complete its metabolic process.

During the practice of nutritional starvation, a minimal amount of calories is required. The body needs at least six to eight hundred calories a day to complete its metabolic processes.

Intermittent fasting is one of the most effective, efficient, and cheapest ways to trigger the process of autophagy. I have personally done some research on some of the types of foods that can boost the body's performance during this process.

In this chapter, we will be discussing the necessary foods and nutrients that must not be avoided during the process of nutritional starvation, as well as the foods to avoid.

Will power is highly overrated, this is one of the major reason why so many diets and nutritional discipline's plans fails. Success can only be obtained when we create an environment that makes success easier than failure.

Therefore, eliminating all the junk food from your kitchen is very important for the process, for you to be successful; it's just like 'autophagy' itself, we clean up all the junky old or damaged cells to create space for the new ones. It might be quite a difficult task at the beginning, but you just have to think that it's much more difficult to resist this kind of food when it's right in front of you.

Here's a list of some of the foods that is better to get rid of before the process of autophagy is practiced;

- **Sugary cereals:** These processed foods are highly concentrated with sugar and high-carb nutrients. Such meals with a high level of sugary concentration are capable of increasing the blood sugar level. This makes it difficult for the body to trigger the process of autophagy. All types of processed cereals must be gotten rid of. Natural and non-processed oats are ok.
- **Sugary cakes and confectioneries.**
- **Chocolates:** except for the chocolates that are composed of a minimum of 70% of cocoa's content. Every other type of chocolates should be eliminated.
- **Snacks:** breakfast bars, crisps, and all types of non-natural dried fruits.
- **Sweet tropical foods must also be disposed of.**
- **Flatbreads and crackers should be gotten rid of.**
- **Alcohol must always be avoided at all costs.**

Pitfall prevention!

The practice of nutritional starvation is only a part of the process that promotes or enhances autophagy; it is important to eat very well during the days in which you do not fast as well. People usually get excited about their level of progress when they do not eat for a whole day. This makes them think that it's better to avoid calorie-dense meals and embrace instead all those meals that are low in calories, hoping that this will speed up the process of autophagy. This is a misconception! This approach tends to slow down the process of metabolism in the body. Instead, it is essential to focus on getting a wide range of energy into the body when you don't fast.

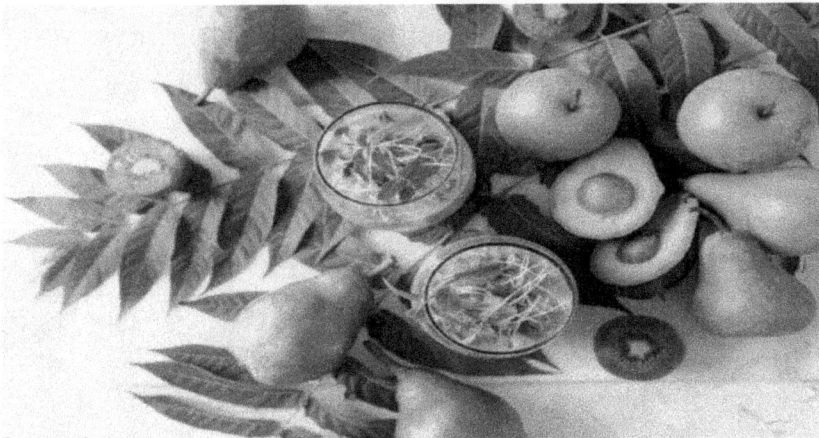

Here is a list of healthy nutrients that can enhance or promote the process of autophagy:

1. MODERATE AMOUNT OF FAT

A moderate quantity of fat, when taken, is satisfying. It must be understood that the body stays full longer after meals that contain a moderate amount of fats than after meals with low or no fat at all. Fat does not, in any way, increase the insulin level of the body. So, it does not contribute to the development of insulin resistance the way foods with a highly concentrated level of carbs would. Therefore, many of the people who have practiced weight-loss plans based on low-fat diets may find it difficult to add fatty foods at the beginning. If you are among them...don't worry! It's only a matter of time, you'll get used to it rapidly.

There are various types of fats, it's important to assume food that contains all of these varieties in order to ensures optimal health and better metabolism in the body.

Below are listed the various types of fats:

- **SATURATED FATS**

    This is the type of fats that contain glycerol and fatty acids. They are found in the fatty portion of foods derived from animals and plants.

    Some of the saturated fatty foods that promote the process of autophagy are;

- ➢ Chicken skin
- ➢ Bacon
- ➢ Pork belly
- ➢ Butter
- ➢ Coconut oils
- ➢ Palm oils
- ➢ Cream
- ➢ Meats
- ➢ Whole milk
- ➢ Cheese
- ➢ Lamb

Saturated fats have been related to heart diseases by medical practitioners and nutritional experts, but consider that there is no definitive evidence to prove these claims. Even if it's true that there is no reason to completely avoid saturated fats, it's also true that it's better to consume them in a moderate quantity and to vary the sources. In fact, there are foods rich in saturated fats healthier than others, which can lower the blood sugar level.

- **MONOSATURATED FATS**

  This type of fat can be found in plants like olives and avocadoes. These types of fats have been linked to lower risk of heart diseases and are capable of enhancing the development and maintenance of the cells. Hence, monosaturated fats are a healthy option and should be incorporated in your meal while practicing nutritional starvation.

Examples of foods that are rich in monosaturated fats are:

> Nuts
> Avocado
> Olive oil
> Sunflower oil
> Peanut oil and butter
> Canola oil
> Safflower oil
> Sesame oil

- **POLYUNSATURATED FATS**

  The polyunsaturated fats are capable to improve in both positive and negative ways, the blood's cholesterol level and to help decrease, if consumed in a moderate quantity, the risk of heart diseases and diabetes.

  Examples of foods with higher amounts of polyunsaturated fats include:

- **Corn oil**
- **Soya bean oil**
- **Safflower oil:** the safflower oil is obtained from the safflower plant; it is a healthy source of fatty acids. It has many health benefits, such as lower cholesterol, it helps to fight against inflammation, it boosts the heart's health and soothes dry skin.
- **Walnuts:** they are a rich source of antioxidants that help reduce the risk of cancer, support weight loss, decrease inflammation, help manage type 2 diabetes, promote a healthy gut, and lower blood pressure.
- **Flax seeds**
- **Flax oils:** this is one of the best sources of omega-3 obtained from plants. It helps to enhance weight loss and reduces the blood sugar level.
- **Salmon**
- **Mackerel**
- **Herring**
- **The albacore tuna**
- **Trout**
- **Sardines**
- **Whole grain wheat**
- **Seaweed**
- **Peanut butter**

- ➤ **Chia seeds**
- ➤ **Turkey breast**

INTRODUCING FAT INTO YOUR DIET

While preparing your meals, olive oil is recommended. You can also use, in small quantities, butter, coconut oil, and other animal fats. The belief that olive oil should only be used while preparing cold meals is a misconception. Olive oil does not have a high smoke point and it's okay to use it for roasting, baking, and even frying.

Avocados are highly rich in healthy fats. It is recommended to make them a regular part of your diet. You can slice it and add it to any of your meals or mash it, creating a cream delicious to spread on the bread. You can use avocados in sauces or in dressings to thicken them. Also, if you are a true fan of avocados, you can include avocado oil in your diet as well. Both avocados and olives are highly rich in monosaturated fats, a fact that makes them a really healthy food choice.

There are also other ways of getting more fats into your diets. Poultry products like whole eggs and low-fat nuts o coconut milk can be easily incorporated into your meals.

2. MODERATE AMOUNT OF PROTEIN

When it comes to protein consumption, a moderate amount of protein is required. Protein is a really important component of the cells; they are important builders and repairers of the body's tissues. Proteins are important in the process of making enzymes, hormones, and other essential chemicals.

However, it's important to know that the consumption of excessive quantities of processed animal products like hot dogs, sausages, and beef has been linked to an increased risk of diabetes, cardiovascular diseases, and cancer.

While undergoing the process of autophagy, it is recommended to get the required dietary proteins from the following sources;

Poultry: poultry products are an important source of protein, especially poultry products like turkey breast, chicken skin, and other birds. They contain less negative fats than other kinds of meats.

Beans: beans are the best source of proteins when compared to the other vegetable sources. They are really rich in fibers that help you feel satisfied for longer hours.

Fish: fish provides the body system with important hearty omega 3 fatty acids.

Nuts: a moderate consumption of nuts like almonds, walnuts and hazelnuts is recommended. They are rich sources of protein for the body while it is experiencing a diet.

Whole grains: A small portion of whole wheat bread provides the body with protein, plus valuable fiber.

Other sources of proteins are; oatmeal, quinoa, lentils, black beans, lean meats, milk, cheese, yogurts, tofu, shrimps, and macadamia oil.

3. NON-STARCHY VEGETABLES

Since we aim to lower the insulin level in the body while fasting, it would be a bad idea to eat a lot of heavy-carb foods, such as potatoes, rice, white bread, and other starches. It's better to eat low-carb foods, like non-starchy vegetables and fruits.

It's highly recommended to eat leafy greens too, like; salad greens, mustard greens, bok choy, arugula, and kale. Brassicas like; cauliflower, cabbages, broccoli, Brussels sprouts, and cucumbers.

Other vegetables always recommend are: garlic, onions, carrots, ginger, turmeric, horseradish bell peppers, okra, mustard greens, zucchini, lettuce, spinach, artichokes, eggplants, Swiss chards, asparagus, silverbeet, celery, pumpkin, shallot, eggplant, baby corn, bamboo shoots, Amaranth, sugar snap peas, water chestnuts, yard-long beans, squash, rutabaga, pea pods, leeks, kohlrabi, hearts of palm, collard, jicama, daikon, coleslaw, celery, chicory, parsley, purslane, snow peas, summer squash, rapini and fennel.

Wild mushrooms are also relevant sources of calories and macronutrients.

4. FRUITS

➢ **Avocadoes:** avocadoes are quite different from the other fruits; most fruits contain a high amount of carbs and a low amount of fat, while in avocados we see the opposite. The fat content of avocado is mostly represented by oleic acid, a monosaturated fat that is linked to a reduction in inflammation and to an improvement in the heart condition.

- In addition, avocadoes are loaded with potassium, fiber, and magnesium, a fact that adds a lot to its health benefits

➢ **Coconuts:** Coconuts are especially rich in manganese, which is essential for healthy bones and for the metabolism of proteins which helps in, turn, to form the red blood cells and also to enhance the repair of worn-out tissues or cells. They also contain selenium, which is an important antioxidant able to protect the cells.

➢ Watermelon: this a rich source of vitamin A and vitamin C. it is also a rich source of some important antioxidants like carotenoids, lycopene, and cucurbitacin E.

- Watermelons have been studied for their anti-cancer effects. The intake of lycopene is likely to reduce the risk of cancers of the digestive system, while antioxidants like cucurbitacin E may reduce the risk of tumor growth.

- The consumption of foods that are rich in lycopene can also promote health because of their ability to reduce cholesterol levels and blood pressure.

- Watermelon is the most hydrating fruit; it is made up of about 92% water, which can keep you hydrated while fasting.

➢ **Olives:** this is a source of vitamin E, iron, calcium, and copper. They help to prevent heart diseases, liver damages and have anti-inflammatory effects. Just like avocado, they contain oleic acids, which help to prevent cancer.

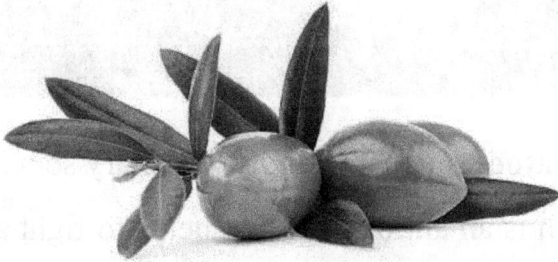

➢ **Raspberries:** they are high in nutrients like vitamin C, vitamin K, vitamin E, potassium, and iron. They contain quercetin and Gallic acids that help to fight cancer and circulatory diseases.

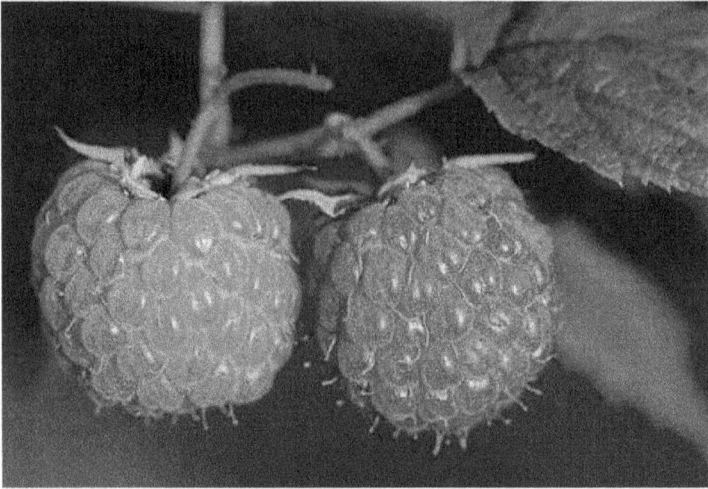

- ➤ **Tomatoes:** they are majorly a dietary source of lycopene, which is an antioxidant that helps to fight and reduce the risk of cancer and heart diseases. They contain nutrients like; folate, potassium, and vitamin C.

- ➤ **Lemons:** This is a very rich citrus fruit, known for its rich vitamin C content. They help in promoting heart health thanks to their ability to lower blood lipids and pressure.

- ➤ **Apples:** they contain an incredibly high amount of fiber, potassium, and vitamin K. they also provide the body with vitamin B. Furthermore, studies have shown that the antioxidants in apples are capable to reduce the risk of cancer, and type 2 diabetes.

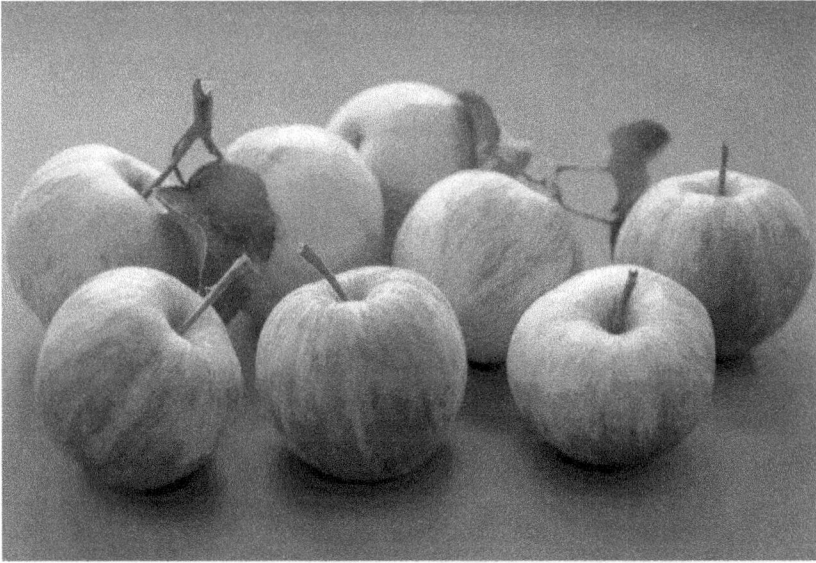

- **Mango:** it's an excellent source of vitamin C. It contains soluble fibers, which are capable of providing numerous health benefits. It's a very strong anti-inflammatory property that may help reduce the risk of diseases.

- **Grapefruit:** this is a good source of vitamins and minerals. They are widely known for their ability to reduce insulin resistance and aid weight loss. It also helps to reduce the cholesterol level and to prevent kidney stones as well.

- **Pineapple:** among all the tropical fruits, pineapple stands out when considering its nutritional contents. It contains a good amount of bromelain, which is a mixture of enzymes known for their inflammatory effects and their ability to digest protein.

- Studies show that the bromelain present in pineapples is capable to protect the body against cancer and tumor formation and growth.

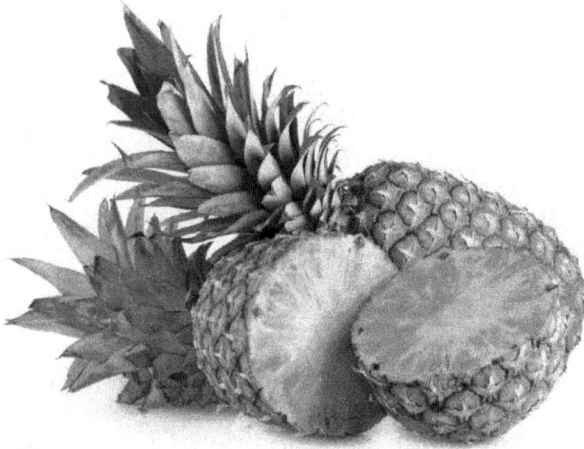

➢ **Strawberries:** they contain nutrients like vitamin C, manganese, potassium, and folate. When compared to other fruits, strawberries have a low glycemic index. Eating them should not cause an increase in blood sugar levels. They help to reduce the risk of chronic diseases.

- They may also help to prevent cancer and tumor growth or formation.

➢ **Blueberries:** they are rich in nutrients like vitamin K, vitamin C, manganese, and fiber. They are believed to contain an impressively positive nutritional profile. They are exceptionally high in their antioxidant level; in fact, they are believed to contain the highest content of antioxidants among fruits. They have a powerful effect on the immune system.

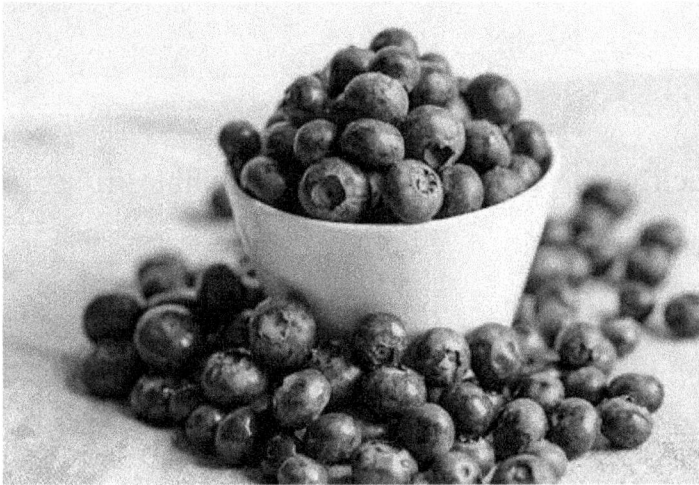

> **Pomegranate:** These are some of the healthiest fruit that you could have. They contain some powerful plant compounds that are responsible for most of their health benefits. They have about three times the antioxidant content that other fruits have. Studies show that they have anti-inflammatory effects able to reduce the risk of cancer.

> **Cranberries:** the cranberries have some impressive health benefits. They are rich in nutrients like manganese, vitamin C, vitamin E, vitamin K, and copper. They help to prevent urinary infections.

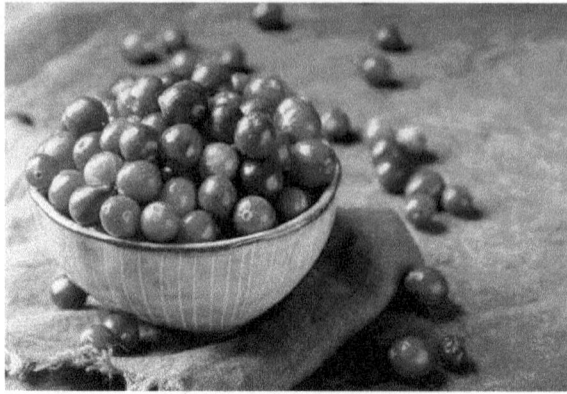

➤ **Blackberries:** these are other incredible fruits, they are packaged with vitamins, minerals, fibers and antioxidants. They provide a significant amount of vitamin C, vitamin K, and manganese. Blackberries also contain some of the antioxidants that reduce inflammation and the arteries' process of aging.

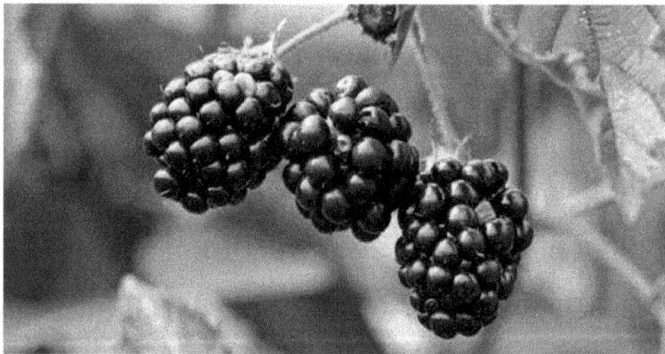

➤ **Oranges:** they are one of the most nutritious fruits; they provide the body with vitamin c and potassium. They are also a rich source of vitamin B. Oranges contain citric acid, that is capable to reduce the risk of stones in the kidneys.

> **Bananas:** they are rich in minerals and vitamins; they are essential for the control of blood sugar's level and for digestive health.

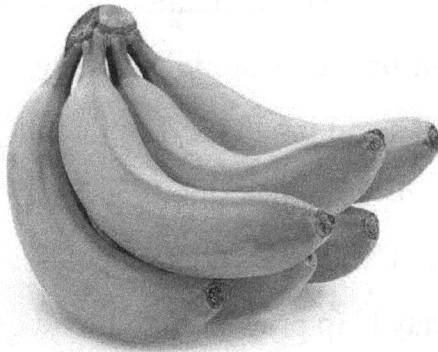

> **Red and purple grapes:** they contain a high content of antioxidants, such as anthocyanin and resveratrol. They help to prevent inflammation.

> **Durian:** they are rich in vitamins B, manganese, folate, copper, and magnesium. They are rich in several healthy plant compounds that function as antioxidants.

> **Pawpaw:** this is a very healthy fruit, rich in nutrients like vitamin c, potassium folate, and vitamin A. This fruit is also rich in antioxidants like lycopene, which helps to prevent cancer.

➤ **Cherries:** this is a rich source of nutrients like potassium, vitamin c, and fiber.

  ▪ They contain some antioxidants like carotenoids and anthocyanin, which help to reduce inflammation and other diseases.

➤ **Cucumber:** they are low in calories but highly rich in vitamins and minerals. They contain antioxidants that may help to reduce the blood sugar level and to lose weight. Cucumbers contain potassium and magnesium that may help prevent high blood pressure.

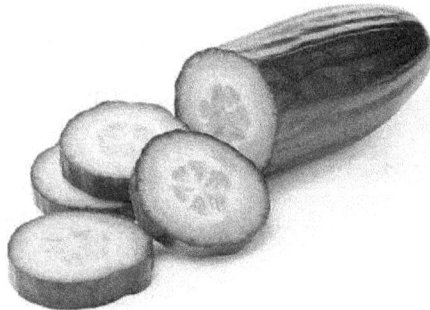

HOW LONG DOES IT TAKE FOR AUTOPHAGY TO KICK IN?

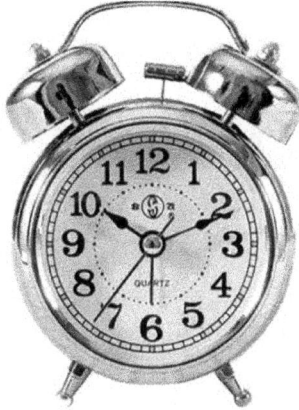

The most notable benefit of autophagy is weight loss and fasting is the process that most triggers it. During the first 24 hours, your body will utilize all of the glycogen available in the liver. After that period, the body will need to run on the nutrients it has stored before. These nutrients can be either proteins or fats.

Autophagy is achieved through the process of intermittent fasting when the glycogen level in the liver is depleted. This usually occurs after **twelve or sixteen** hours into the fasting period. The autophagy rate reaches its peak at this point and then drops after two days, more or less.

Some other researches claim that it could take about 48 to 72 hours of fasting to kick-start or initiate the process of autophagy. This is because the body may enter into ketosis and may start producing ketone bodies before.

Although there are no viable ways to measure autophagy in humans, it can be guessed or estimated by controlling the glucose ketone index and the insulin - glucagon ratio. By doing this, you can estimate when the process of autophagy kicks in.

The moment in which autophagy kicks in for a particular person depends on the nutrient status of the person's system and on the presence of certain nutrients, like amino acids, ketones, and glucose.

Hence, if a person does not consume too many carbs or proteins daily, the process of autophagy is expected to occur faster.

The more carbs or proteins you eat, the longer you have to fast to get into autophagy. Consuming more quantity of calories than required in fact, will increase the number of molecules that needs to be burnt before that autophagy can start to act.

CHAPTER SIX
COMMON MISTAKES AND
MISCONCEPTIONS

Autophagy has gained a lot of popularity in the last period since researchers have discovered that it helps the body with a multitude of benefits. Our quest for comfortability and a stress-free life has led us to a wide range of discoveries. In the dawn of humanity, when only survival, through hunting and gathering, was important, the man was able to construct a balance within its social-cultural environment. Today, we face many diseases that have the capacity to complicate human life in a new way. This is why we are constantly looking for advanced information and strategies able to put and maintain our body in the right shape. Autophagy is one of these mechanisms able to improve our quality of life and fasting and other stressful activities do accelerate it to a perfect cleansing level.

Many persons have developed in the last period a lot of interest for fasting— even if fasting is something that is in practice since the emergence of man, it's not something new; it is also associated with religious beliefs. Christians, Jews; l, Muslims during Ramadan, Buddhists, and other religions honor and appreciate fasting in their realities. All the recent interest in fasting gave autophagy popularity and a lot has been said, true and not true. It's important for me to talk about some of the common mistakes and myths about autophagy. First of all, it's important to say that the majority of people typically fast in order to lose weight but, the actions of autophagy are mostly focused on the protection of the body against infectious diseases. The basic idea of autophagy is simple to understand: the absence of external sources of food makes the body able to eat itself, by recycling and renew old parts and enabling a new and healthier version of the self to come into existence. Furthermore, autophagy helps protects against diseases like cancer, dementia, skin diseases, and many others, as discussed in the previous chapters. Fasting and reducing the intake of calories tend to reduce weight and to slow down the process of aging.

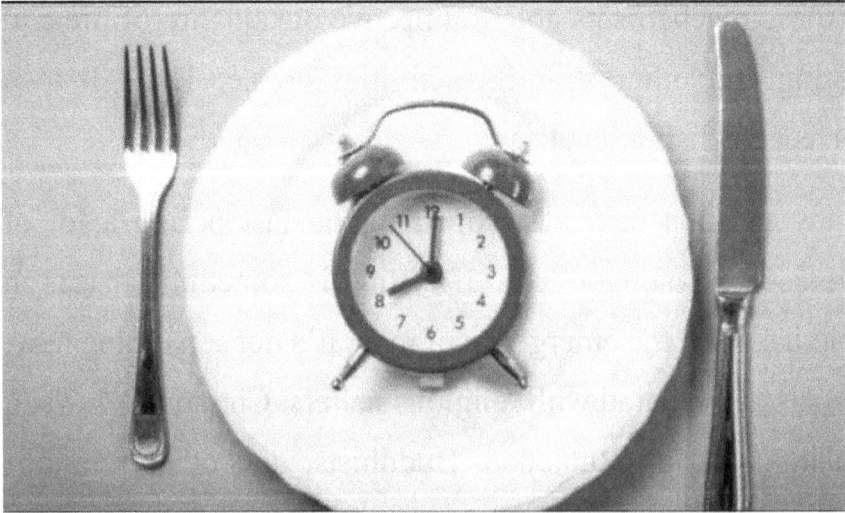

In any case, you have also to keep in mind that this field is relatively new and a lot of things are yet to be discovered. I'm simply discussing with you the logic that stands behind what autophagy is: it is the process that allows the human's body to burn down the old and to build, out of the ashes, new and more effective components. In this field, few are the researches conducted on humans, most of them are based on mice and yeast.

In a research done on mice, it was discovered that it takes 24 hours before autophagy can occur, but mice metabolism does not necessarily correspond to human metabolism. In an interview, Jason Fung, the researcher, suggested that autophagy, in which "your body will take the oldest, junkiest proteins and burn them for energy, will happen probably in the later stages of a long fast — somewhere around 20 to 24 hours, is my guess, and it probably reaches a maximal activity somewhere around 32 hours. Again, this is my best guess." Caloric restriction and fasting are the best-known ways of promoting autophagy in the human body as well.

THE TANGLED —MISCONCEPTION

First, you should understand that fasting is different from autophagy itself. The first deals with weight control, slower aging and is able to trigger autophagy, which protects the body against diseases and activate mechanisms of reparation. You should note that autophagy is already a physiological part of cells function, activated in all the occasions in which unwanted or unnecessary material is produced, in order to avoid the body's breakdown or illness. Be aware that there are misconceptions about what are the diseases that autophagy can help proffer a perfect cure; the information available is a little bit confusing. As I said earlier, the majority of the researches done on autophagy is conducted on mice and the results are not necessarily applicable to men. In recent times, some studies have proved to us that autophagy can help fight infectious diseases, regulate inflammation and increase the immune system's efficiency. It is also said that increased longevity could be associated too with the process of autophagy, BUT this connection seems to be a bit blurry and not clear. In any case, it is true that it has been proved to be effective in mice, it puts them in better shape and increases their lifespan.

Now, researchers are trying to better understand how fasting can help fighting cancer or, at least, its basic interaction with it. The findings are still a bit confusing. Notice that some of the studies conducted have discovered that autophagy can cause cancer to be stronger, with a high resistance to radiation. It seems that autophagy can both act as a tumor suppressor or promoter, depending on the circumstances. Autophagy is a **double-edged sword**—it owns the ability to heal and, at the same time, can cause some adverse effects. Its positive and negative role in cancer makes it difficult for us to be able to applicate it properly in cancer therapy.

There are many concerns about the fact that too much fasting, that can actually control weight, could be dangerous among those persons with cancer. Recently, nevertheless, the 2016 JAMA Oncology study conducted on women with breast cancer has discovered that those who fasted for more than 13 hours a day had lower rates of cancer's recurrence.

I must state that a plethora of studies is ongoing in order to unclad the dark veil that still covers the face of autophagy, so that speculation could stop, and a universal theory could be established.

You should note that autophagy could prevent and also mitigate serious injuries but, be aware that fasting, in the majority of cases, is not good for underweight people, young lads, and older people.

THE MYTHS ASSOCIATED WITH AUTOPHAGY

Here, I want to address the most common myths and objections associated with autophagy, so that you can do it safely, and effectively.

- **Autophagy causes muscle wasting:** it is important to state clearly that there are two types of energy that the human body stores, which are **fat** and **sugar**. The proteins, that make up your muscles, are not used by the body for energy production during a brief fasting. The proteins in the muscles are extremely inefficient and it takes a lot of energy for the body to break down the muscles. I can support this statement by calling your attention back to the time when men where based on hunting and gathering and continuously fought in order to survive. If the energy in their muscles would have been wasted because of hunger before they could have provided another meal, that would have made them susceptible to other predators. Their survival was possible because they could still use the fat stored as energy when there was a temporary shortage of food. It's totally wrong to think that our beloved muscles are the first to be weakened during a fast.

- **When I finally eat, I will rapidly become fatter than before:** it is simple, you won't get fatter. When you finally eat, after a fast, your body will need to replenish its stores of glycogen in the liver and the muscles first, it won't store fat immediately. So, the perfect answer to this misconception is "No". The human body typically stores about 2000 calories in the liver, and this is the simplest energy source for the body to access and use. Therefore, being the beautifully efficient machine that your body is, it will likely want to replenish up its easiest food source first. When and only when your glycogen stores are full, your body will start sending excess calories to the fat cells for storage.

- **Autophagy means malnourishment:** over time, this common belief has led many people into confusion and disagreement. During fasting, no new food is introduced into the system and there is a high reduction in calories—this is the basic explanation of fasting. There is a belief that during fasting, a lot of energy is lost and malnourishment is inevitable, likewise a loss of essential vitamins and minerals, leaving us malnourished, weak and depleted. During a fast that lasts less than 24 hours (often called intermittent fasting), there is no need to be worried about a loss in vitamins or minerals. All the vitamins and energy lost during a day of fasting are rapidly replenished, while for any fast longer than 24 hours it is important to always supplement with sodium, potassium, and magnesium. This is because, in a fasted state, with the drop of the insulin levels, your kidneys will release the water in excess and, with it, a lot of vital micronutrients that we need for cellular function. In any case, this loss of nutrients is not enough to make you malnourished.

- **Breakfast is the most legit meal of the day:** it's being many years that, our mind has been fed with the lie that breakfast is the most important meal of the day, but let's tell the truth, usually, we wake up, we don't actually feel hungry. We eat early in the morning because we have been told to do so, we accept the belief that it's healthier without questioning it. You should note that throughout the night, our body has been fasting until we wake up, in order to determine whether you are hungry or not, you should drink a tall glass of water. You will discover that what you call "hunger" disappears, it was a mere psychological illusion of our mind. In essence, you should eat when you're really hungry. The most important meal of the day is when you break your fast. If you are doing short, daily fasts, this typically happens around lunchtime.

- **Autophagy is unhealthy:** this is a lie; autophagy is good for the body, even if it's true that our knowledge in this field is not complete. Many persons ask themselves: "why will I have to fast when I can secure myself a good meal?" the simple answer is that you're fasting because you want to protect your body against yourself.

- **You attain autophagy within 24 hours:** the truth is, it is very difficult to get a magnificent boost in autophagy within this time frame. Physical activity, done while fasting, can help you get it faster, but actually, A 17 hours fast might not be able to get you any autophagy activated. You should note that you don't start to fast right after a meal's intake because the body needs to digest all the nutrients introduced, a process that takes at least 4-5 hours, depending on what kind of foods you ate. For example, foods like, fiber, vegetables, proteins and fat take a longer time to digest. The real fast commences after 5-6 hours after the meal's intake, before that, you're still in the fed state and you're burning the calories that you have just eaten.

- **Autophagy means starvation:** autophagy is not starvation. When you become unable to eat or consume exogenous calories, you reach the condition called starvation. Every human has body fat, even an extreme lean man has from 40 to about 50000 calories stored, that can help him survive for weeks, if not months. Under a condition of energy deprivation, the body is forced to recycle its weaker components, a fact that wouldn't occur while eating. Fast and autophagy do not mean starvation, they only indicate a state in which the human body goes through a process of self-renewal and general healing that cannot occur while food is consumed. Thinking of autophagy as starvation is definitely not correct. On the contrary, this process is one of the best things you can do to help your body to survive longer.

- **Autophagy consumes loose skin:** This is relatively true, but only to a certain extent. It is widely believed that autophagy can eat up loose skin and tighten it up after losing a bunch of weight. Although autophagy might be responsible for slowing down the aging of the human skin, it is not able to eat up loose skin and wrinkles. It only supports the processes that keep the skin more elastic and able to tighten up faster. In the cases of extreme overweight, autophagy and fasting might play a role in the prevention of the appearance of excess loose skin but still, it's inevitable that you will experience some loose skin after losing a significant amount of weight.

- **Autophagy cannot be triggered while you consume meat:** It is believed that consuming any kind of meat or food with a higher protein level will never help you to get autophagy activated and will speed up the process of aging. When it comes to autophagy, the frequency on which you eat is the most important thing to take care of. If you eat 3 times a day and never fast any longer than 24 hours, then you still won't gain significant autophagy's activation even if you restrict your proteins and meat intake. Furthermore, carbohydrates and insulin also stop autophagy, that means that even a fully plant-based vegan diet won't give you an increase in autophagy if you're eating too frequently.

- **Coffee halt autophagy:** No. Drinking coffee does not halt autophagy; instead, it helps and promotes autophagy and ketosis. The polyphenols contained in your coffee are able to stimulate the activation of autophagy. Caffeine's ketone bodies can feed part of your brain and, by doing so, reduce its glucose requirement significantly. It also promotes lipolysis, the burning of fatty acids, which enables to lower the insulin level, to raise AMPK, and boost ketones. To have all these positive effects from coffee, you'd have to drink it black without any milk, cream, or sugar—since all kinds of sweeteners raise insulin and halt the fasting process. Milk and dairy especially raise IGF-1, which activates mTOR. Notice that even zero-calorie sweeteners raise insulin via the cephalic phase response that prepares insulin in the gut.

- **Exercise can stop autophagy:** it is the other way around; exercise cannot stop autophagy; instead, it increases it. Exercise induces autophagy. Next to fasting, exercising and working out are the best thing to do in order to increase autophagy, as well as to promote general health and a perfect body. The best thing to do would be to combine and practice them both consistently.

- **Your brain regularly needs the supply of dietary glucose:** it sounds surprising, but some persons claimed that the human brain needs a constant supply of dietary glucose. If you do not eat carbs every few hours, your brain might not function properly. They based their argument on the belief that the human brain can only use glucose for fuel, but this is not true. Your body can always produce glucose whenever it is needed via a process called **gluconeogenesis**. Ketone bodies can feed parts of your brain, reducing its glucose requirement significantly. However, some people report feeling fatigued or shaky when they don't eat for a while. If this applies to you, you should consider keeping snacks on hand or eating more frequently, in order to avoid any problem.

- **Skipping breakfast can make you fat:** most people believe that breakfast is the most important meal of the day. Hence, skipping breakfasts will result in excessive hunger, cravings, and weight gain. Studies have proven that breakfast does not primarily affect your body weight, although there may be some variability. The study even showed that the people who lose weight over a long period of time tend to eat breakfast. In summary, breakfast can be of great importance for many people, but not essential to one's health. It's already proven that people can skip it and remain healthy without any negative consequences.

- **Fasting leaves the body in a starvation mode:** one of the most common arguments against the intermittent fasting as a process of triggering autophagy is that it puts the body in a starvation mode, that can shut down the metabolism and prevent the body from burning fats. While it is true that a long period of weight loss can reduce the number of calories that the body burns over time, there is no proof or scientific backing that intermittent fasting causes a great reduction in the calories burned by the body when compared to other weight loss methods. It's just the opposite, intermittent fasting is capable of increasing the metabolic rates of the body. This is due to the increase in the blood's norepinephrine's level, which stimulates the rate at which metabolism occurs.

In fact, studies have shown that fasting for about 48 hours may boost the rate of metabolism from about 3 to 14%. However, if you fast for a longer period of time, the effects can be reversed.

- **Autophagy can lead to loss of muscles:** there is a widespread belief that the process of autophagy enables the body to burn muscles for fuel. There is no scientific evidence that this happens when undergoing autophagy, especially when triggered by intermittent fasting.

On the contrary, studies show that intermittent fasting is better for maintaining muscle mass. In fact, intermittent fasting is very popular among many bodybuilders, who believe that it helps maintain the muscles alongside with a low percentage of body fat.

Autophagy has generated a significant amount of false beliefs in the last period of time, we have highlighted a bunch of these generally pervaded myths. The majority of these myths are not true as we have already seen. I'd like to underline again, that fasting does not have the same function of autophagy, they are not the same thing.

All the information provided here is to help you debunk fallacies associated with the concept of autophagy. In any case, it is really important that you consult your health practitioner before you jump into autophagy and remember: knowledge is the heart of success.

CHAPTER SEVEN
SIDE EFFECTS OF AUTOPHAGY

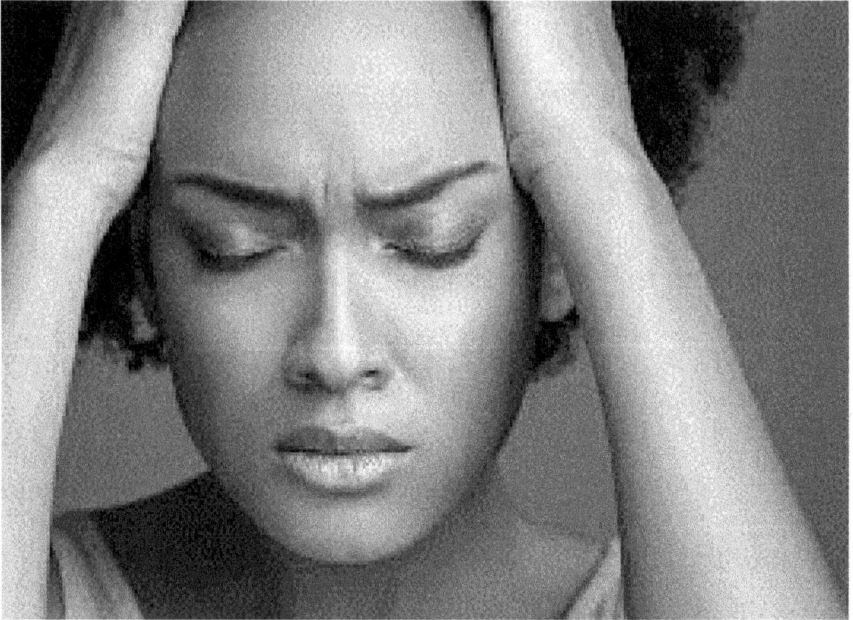

This book would be incomplete without proper insight into the possible side effects that could be experienced in an attempt to trigger the process of autophagy. You surely have already read about the benefits associated with autophagy in the previous chapters, its ability to reduce inflammation, to improve digestion, to reduce bloating, to increase mental clarity, just to cite some benefits. You are ready to give it a try but first, you should consider diligently the side effects that you may likely experience during your journey into autophagy. You have to consider that it takes a while for our body to adjust itself to new changes—especially the extreme ones. So, whoever is prepared and willing to undergo the process of autophagy should take into consideration that it's probable to experience some side effects at first while practicing fasting.

Although these side effects might be very difficult at the beginning, as time goes on you will get used to them and it will become easier; simply, you'll know before what you will experience and you'll find an excellent way to deal with it. In any case, as we said earlier, whatever changes in your diet you want to apply, including the ones that involve autophagy's stimulation, always consult your doctor first, for safer and better results. We gathered some inevitable effects that may be experienced while undergoing the process of autophagy. Among them are:

- **Real Hunger:** this usually happens at the beginning of the autophagy's process. A lot of people reported experiencing real hunger during the first phase of the fasting period. We have tried to differentiate between **"hunger"** and **"real hunger"** because the first might be psychological and can be eased with a tall glass of water, while the second makes you feel really depleted and your stomach intensively requests a meal to ease the disturbance. You should get a clear definition of hunger in your head before you start. People who consume about 5 to 6 meals a day have a higher chance to experience this side effect. The hormone in our body, which is responsible for making us feel **'hungry'**, is called **ghrelin**. It typically reaches the zenith at breakfast, lunch, and dinner time and is partially regulated by our food intake. At the beginning of a fast, it will take a great willpower to overcome this sensation of 'hunger.' The first three / six days of intermittent fasting might look terrible and unbearable, but be confident, a time in which you won't feel so hungry will soon come. Furthermore, in the beginning phase of a fast, you should drink more water, this will help you to divert your mind from the sensation of great-hunger.

- **Headache:** as your body is trying to adjust itself to this new eating pattern, you are likely to experience some dull headaches that may occur randomly, this is very common. In this case too, it will help to drink more water. With time, your body will get used to this new eating schedule, but, in any case, it's always better to try to remain as much stress-free as possible.

- **Serious cravings:** this is a psychological effect common for us, humans; we tend to crave the things that we haven't consumed over a long period of time. When you start fasting, you should expect your body to crave junk foods like ice cream, pizza, chocolate, and other goodies you do consume on a "normal" diet. The best thing to do is doing whatever you can, in order to not think about food, and be sure to indulge your desires a little during your feeding window.

- **You may feel cold:** this usually happens while fasting, the body system automatically becomes more sensitive to cold when the blood sugar level is reduced. Cold fingers and toes are common among the people who are fasting. You can deal with the cold by taking hot tea, wearing a sweatshirt, taking a warm shower, staying away from cold liquids, and wearing extra layers of clothes, amongst others.

- **Irritation:** this happens when you go into the more complex phases of the autophagy process. You tend to feel angry or slighted irritated. You should know that this is not usually your fault, it's not due to your own will; this happens because you start to react to some sort of pressure that you are experiencing internally. The best thing that you can do for yourself is to avoid the situations and people that may likely make you angrier and focus more on the things that make you happy. Just live free with those that can put a smile on your face. This is good advice in general, by the way, valid also when you are not fasting!

- **Consuming lots of food during your feeding window:** if you are new to the process of autophagy, you are likely to eat uncontrollably when you start to eat again after a period of food deprivation. You'll want to consume more food because you'll know that there is no restriction in calories, so you'll probably exaggerate at first. You may be extremely hungry by the time your fasting window will end, this hunger will make you eat really fast and you will end up eating way more than you usually would. Try to be aware of this possible behavioral pattern and opt for healthier options instead, like a grilled chicken and a salad: pleasure and sweetness will overwhelm your mind.

- **Low Energy:** during autophagy, your body consumes less energy because of the low intake of carbs. Your body does not produce the constant fuel that you experience when you eat regularly, so you should expect to feel a little sluggish and tired during the first couple of weeks. Try to keep your day as relaxed as possible, so that you can exert a lesser amount of energy. You might also want to give your workouts a break or do light exercises like walking or yoga. Getting extra sleep may also help.

- **You can always quit:** start your journey at the right time, when you are ready, all these highlighted effects can look at first very bad. They do usually occur when you are a beginner and usually last for the first 1 to 3 weeks. Don't go too hard on yourself; autophagy is not a process meant to cause harm to the human body but to make life a comfortable place to reside. If you are the type of person that normally eats 6 meals, don't start to eat 2 meals suddenly, give your body the time to adapt. After a while, autophagy will become natural and healthy for you.

- **You are the only person who can communicate with your body:** you should note that some persons are restricted from taking autophagy. People with diabetes, pregnant women, nursing mothers, and children are not allowed to practice autophagy because of the side effects associated with it. If fasting is interfering with your ability to keep up with your responsibilities, or if it's making you develop an unhealthy obsession with food, you may need to cut your fast shorter and eat earlier than you planned, or you may need to stop fasting altogether. If you have any concerns or issues, it's always a good idea to consult your doctor to avoid any kind of problems.

- **Unstable blood sugar levels:** during the process of autophagy, the blood's sugar level may rise or fall, depending on the intake of carbohydrates. Both high blood sugar levels and extremely low blood sugar levels are bad. As recently discussed in the previous chapters, autophagy can be triggered by intermittent fasting. Be aware that when the period of fasting is too long, it triggers a negative effect on your body system. Studies have shown that intermittent fasting can lead to a hypoglycemic state, which throws your body systems out of balance. Hence, a prolonged pattern of skipping meals and nutritional starvation will lead to chronic weakness.

- **Hormonal imbalance:** some of the diseases that have an hormonal imbalance as their major cause, like the PCOS, usually request balanced and regular meals for their cure. Don't underestimate the importance of hormonal imbalances, they can put the body system in a constant state of struggle.

- **The acidic level of the body may become imbalanced:** studies and researches from various scientists and nutritionists have shown that the best type of diet to follow is the alkaline diet. A high alkaline diet can help you contrast the acidic effects of certain foods and can help you lose weight. Long-time nutritional starvation may leave the body in an acidic state and an acidic body is an easy prey for diseases. Acidity can also stimulate migraines. If the body is unable to maintain a healthy balance, your efforts will only result in an unhealthy loss of weight.

- **Heartburns:** the process of nutritional starvation during autophagy may lead to heartburn. The lack of food results in the reduction of the acidic level in the stomach. The stomach acid is responsible for the digestion of food and the destruction of bacteria. During the fasting period, thinking of food can trigger the brain to tell the stomach to produce more acid, which leads to experience heartburn.

DETOX EFFECTS: WHAT TO EXPECT

Before you step into a deep detox process, you should note that it has side effects that might seem very serious to our body systems. Being aware of this is by itself an important part of detoxification, it will help you alleviate your worries. The detox explained here is designed to help the body detoxify toxins out of its systems. The detox process starts with dry fasting (no intake of food and drinks at all). After that, a strict diet of water, fresh fruits and vegetable juices, raw fruits and vegetables is applied. You should note that, sometimes, the detox diet can include herbs and other natural supplements. Furthermore, toxins can be targeted by removing some specific items from your daily routine, like for example caffeine, nicotine, and refined sugars.

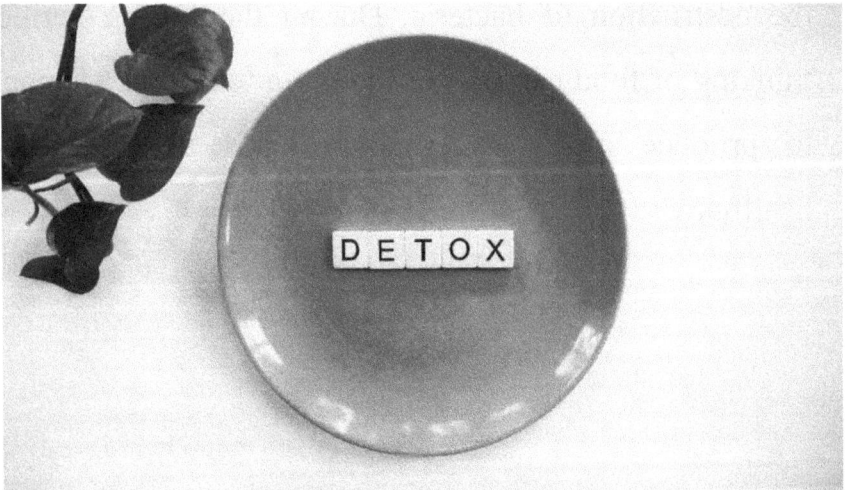

Most detox processes can be self-managed. Obviously, medically supervised detox programs are put in place for alcohol and opiate addicts; this is the essential first step needed to address those that have a chronic dependency. This kind of detox should be done with medical attention, it should never be self-managed. You should note that when you're on a detox phase, you could experience heavy side effects that can manifest themselves in the form of headaches. During these side effects, your body is simply reacting to the fact that items that are regularly introduced in the body are missing. Besides headaches, there are a bunch of effects that you can experience during a detox diet. For example:

- **You will experience fatigue and disrupted sleep:** when you stimulate the body to purge out toxins, it requires a greater internal workload than normal. This creates fatigue and sometimes disrupts our beloved sleep routine. Expect to feel more tired and try to respond to this sensation by resting more than you normally do. Take naps when you can and get to bed at the very latest by 10 pm, it will help. Go to bed with a plan to get a complete 8 hours of sleep at night. When you are sleeping, your body can work efficiently at repairing and cleansing itself.

Scheduling more rest than you are usually used to, will help you ensure that you will get enough downtime even if your sleep is disturbed. Do not add any additional task than normal because it will make your tiredness worse. Stick to light exercises—but don't overdo them. Remember, any stress of whatsoever, either physical, emotional, or mental, is bad for the body.

- **Headache:** experiencing a dull and prolong headache is inevitable. Many people have reported that they witnessed a headache while detoxing. The appearance of headaches during the process of detoxification is prevalent in the afternoon and in the evening. Headache is one of the giant symptoms of detoxification. You witness this side effect because you change your daily routine, and you most likely halt some bad habits such as artificial sugars intake, drinking alcohol, high amounts of caffeine intake and smoking.

- **Nausea:** changing your lifestyle or trying to adapt to something new, will require the body system to make some adjustments. The introduction of herbs and other supplementary nutrients may cause little nausea. The perfect way to avoid nausea is through hydration, adequate relaxation, and the intake of capsules with a little quantity of food and water. In a few days, you will stop experiencing nausea. If instead it proceeds to vomit and nervous breakdown, something else may be going on. Consult your doctor.

- **Cravings:** when detoxing, there is a huge chance that you will desire foods and other things that you haven't consume for a long period of time, especially junk food will have a great power of attraction on you. Changing your diet and lifestyle practices can create a situation of temporary withdrawal. This will most definitely trigger cravings associated with those areas you have changed or eliminated. For example, if you do consume alcoholic drinks every day, it will be difficult for you to spend two or five days without consuming it. In the beginning, this will look like hell because your body will be seriously "needing" it. Even pictures do help trigger cravings. So, stay away from anything that can worsen the situation.

- **Frequent urination:** over time, a large number of persons have reported to experience more frequent urination; this happens because urine is one of the ways through which the body system gets rid of its toxins. Furthermore, some of the herbs taken to clean the body may be diuretic and can cause you to urinate continually and even to experience bowel movements. It is a shock for the digestive system to suddenly deal with different herbs, nutrients, whole new foods, and fresh meals that are different from the previous foods it was used to process. That is why hydration and consumption of whole nutrient-rich food diets are of great importance for the body. Taking multivitamins will help the body to replenish its lost nutrients.

- **You will be obsessed with food:** during the deep phases of detoxification, you will probably only think about food. Various types of meals will frequently pop up in your mind. It might get hard for you at this stage and it's better for you not to be in the presence of people eating or preparing normal meals. The best strategy is to try as much as possible to stay away from anything that can trigger cravings and hunger.

- **You will later look amazing:** after the great difficulty and suffering has passed, you will notice how amazingly great you will feel. There is a reward for every tough minute you have witnessed. You will feel so good that you almost won't remember the tough times you have witnessed before.

HOW TO DEAL WITH DETOX

We have highlighted the side effects that you might witness when you start a detox process. It is now essential to give some important guidelines to help you combat the side effects and the other problems that you might encounter. Over time, addiction has been only linked to the people who have problems with alcohol, nicotine, drugs, and gambling. But in reality, the term "addiction" is valid for a wider range of situations. Addiction interferes with people's financial stability; addiction can destroy your well-being. When addiction gets to this stage, you should look for help and start to detoxify yourself from any kind of toxins present in your system. You should also know that withdrawal symptoms are very unpleasant because the body has been taught to live in the wrong way for a long period of time. A lot of people are not aware that there are a lot of things to be aware of in order to make the detox process bearable and cool. A bit of preparation will make it easier and even enjoyable.

In this section, we will help you know what to expect when going through the detox process and we will help you fight the side effects. Keep always in mind that the detox process is a way to remove all the toxins from the body. These toxins might include drugs, alcohol, and sugar and should be done under strict medical advice.

We have now organized a list of things you can do to contrast the unpleasant things you can experience during a detox process:

- **Consider medical assessment:** assessment should be considered to improve the process. Try to check out into detox centers; this will help determine your total health condition and how severe your addiction is. After the completion of your assessment, it will be decided if you'll need any medication during your initial detox. You will be certainly provided with all the information needed regarding the type of supplements you will need to stay healthy. Detox doesn't always exclude the intake of all medications; some non-addictive medicines can help reduce the common withdrawal associated with detox. Examples of these drugs are nonsteroidal anti-inflammatory drugs (NSAIDs) like ibuprofen and aspirin for pain, anti-anxiety medications such as SSRIs and topical analgesics. All these medicines should be taken only after doctor's prescription to secure a good result.

- **Therapies and counseling should be considered:** while going through detoxification physically, it will be also useful to consider attending physical meetings and counseling at the detox centers. Furthermore, at the centers, additional help and treatments are available. The meetings and the counseling will help you know that you are not alone in the journey. Lots of information will be made available for you, like a guide to 12-Step programs and counseling programs outside of the treatment center itself. Some of the available meetings are focused on addictions, while others cover mainly topics like stress management, family counseling, and training in a different variety of skills. It is important for you to not concentrate too much on your physical withdrawal and to take part in meetings and sessions to obtain a good result.
- **The physical detox:** we are all already aware that detox can involve days of physical discomfort and difficulty to achieve the objectives you set for yourself. You can take detoxification slowly or use medication to help your body adjust safely. If you choose to experience your detox process in a center, you're guaranteed a 24 hours strict supervision.

- **Nutrition:** every one that experiences a detox phase underlines the importance of nutrition during the process. You might be tempted to go back to junk food, but keep in mind that your body is in a deep process of repairing itself. What it needs is healthy, reparative foods, that facilitate its journey towards health. You will need to regain all the nutrients that went lost because of the withdrawal symptoms, like constant vomiting, diarrhea, and severe tiredness. Good nutrition will help you flush out faster every addictive substance that your fat cells stored. Try to make a good meal plan before starting a detox. It doesn't only promote health in general, it promotes stability during detox too, giving to you less possibilities to think about cravings. Eating healthy foods in fact, can also boost in a positive way your mood by triggering the natural release of endorphins and increase the energy in the body. Never stop drinking a lot of water and taking vitamins to help the body sustain the detox process.

- **Other available treatment:** there are many available treatments that you can use during your detox process. They can reduce pain and help relaxation. I'm talking about treatments like massages, acupuncture, yoga, meditation, breathing exercises, art-based therapy, and pet therapy. Although they might not be strictly created to be part of an addiction's treatment, you have to consider that anything that gives you happiness and provides a good distraction during the detox period is very important. You should take part in several positive activities during the withdrawal process. If you don't do so, into depression, which you can easily fall into depression problems.

- **Exercise will help:** a moderate physical exercise can help the body to be in good shape and eliminate physical and psychological withdrawal symptoms typical of the detox phase. Although while struggling with addiction, you might not want to pay attention to exercise, which includes strength or aerobic endurance, planning a moderate sport routine can help improve heart health, lung capacity, muscle tone, and digestive performance. When you put yourself into physical activity, you will enjoy benefits like reduction in body fats and overall weight, lower risk of having cardiovascular diseases, lower risk of type 2 diabetes and metabolic syndrome, reduced risk of some types of cancer, and stronger bones and muscles.

- **Music is life:** you might have already heard the sentence "Music is life"…and, in the detox process, it is quite true. Music has an important role to be played here, it is able in fact to make you lively and happy. The power of music will help you ease the withdrawal symptoms. In rehabilitation programs, music therapy may include you writing a song, learning to play instruments, engaging in singalongs with other people and other approaches to actively engaging with music. Music can help reduce the likelihood of relapse.

We have provided all the necessary information that concerns the effects of autophagy so that you can step into it consciously and fully aware. It is of great importance for you, understand that consulting your doctor or physician will help you understand what is good and what might look dangerous for your health. So, join the world of great explorations and live a life free from illness and unacceptable body's breakdowns. Utilize these words as a guide to become a man able to start a journey towards liberation and self-actualization.

FREQUENTLY ASKED QUESTIONS
ABOUT AUTOPHAGY

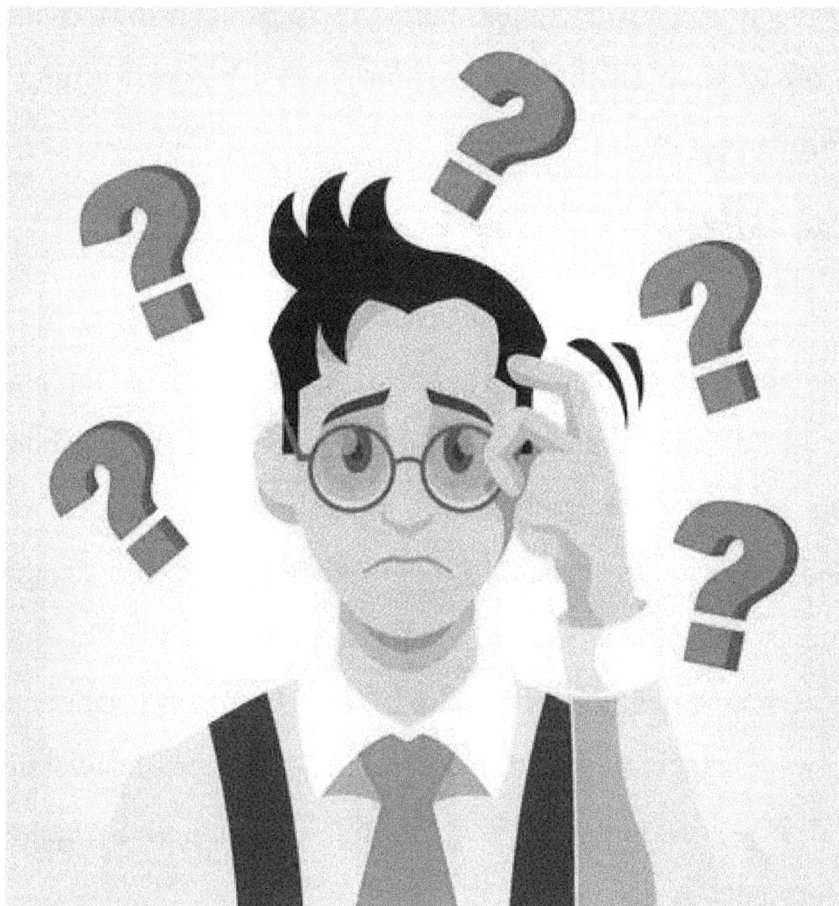

In this book, we have discussed one of the most powerful, and almost magical, thing that our body can do for itself: autophagy. As we have seen, autophagy is not so difficult to understand and I hope that I gave you all the necessary information to apply it in the previous chapters. Although it has been proven to be a true superpower, autophagy has generated some concern across the world and many questions have been frequently asked. We will try to answer them in this section. I always recommend you to be open-minded and to try to have all the information needed before forming a definitive opinion about it.

Can autophagy heal cancer completely?

Answer: Although some studies have proven that autophagy could help weaken and confuse cancer in the human body and give a significant help when applied in traditional medicine's treatments, like chemotherapy, there are other studies that have proven that autophagy can have both positive and negative effects on cancer. This hazy connection between cancer and autophagy has led to many controversies and it's still not sure if it should be applied in cancer treatments or not.

o **Is autophagy good for our health?**

Answer: autophagy helps our body in many ways. It's able to optimize our organism so that it can live longer and in better health. It helps the body to destroy its damaged cells so that new and healthier components can be built.

o **Can autophagy occur if I don't fast that long?**

Answer: Yes, autophagy can occur, but it is difficult to measure it— a fact that makes it not easy for us to calculate the rate at which it occurs in our body. You should take note that autophagy occurs regularly within certain organisms like humans, mice, and yeast, and some factors can help accelerate the rate at which it occurs, like, for example, fasting and other forms of stress (exercise).

o **Is autophagy just mere speculation?**

Answer: Autophagy is not just mere speculation, although our knowledge in this field is still incomplete and it just gained popularity in recent times. If autophagy was only speculation, we wouldn't have any practical knowledge about it. Today, our knowledge is not complete because there are fewer studies conducted on man. However, the studies conducted on mice have shown us that autophagy is not speculation at all. A 2016 JAMA Oncology study on women with breast cancer found that those who fasted for more than 13 hours a day had lower rates of cancer recurrence in their life. Many studies on autophagy are ongoing, soon we'll have more data about it.

o **Can autophagy be harmful?**

Answer: Autophagy has been described as "a double-edged sword" because of its ability to both palliate and escalate injury. Fasting itself can cause, when done incorrectly, negative effects. That's why you should always applicate these mechanisms carefully and under medical supervision.

o **Can I drink water during autophagy?**

Answer: studies have shown that water fasting too has the ability to activate autophagy. Although It seems also to be able to lower the risk of some chronic diseases, human studies on water fasting are still limited and, hence, the results incompleted.

o **How long does it take for the body to get into ketosis during autophagy?**

Answer: Studies show that it takes approximately 2 to 4 days for the body to enter into ketosis when the food intake is lower than 50 grams of carbs per day. In any case, be aware that it may take a longer period of time in some people, depending on some factors like; physical activity level, age, metabolism, and previous diets habits.

o **Does the intake of coffee stop autophagy?**

Answer: the intake of caffeine has some effects on autophagy; a little quantity of caffeine intake in the early hours of the day may increase that valuable recycling time as you fast. Studies have shown that both the normal and the decaffeinated brands of coffee can cause a rapid occurrence of autophagy in lab rats (from about 1 to 4 hours after the coffee was consumed).

o **Is being in ketosis safe?**

Answer: the process of ketosis occurs when a low or no carbs diet is consumed and molecules called ketones are produced, increasing their level in the bloodstream. Many studies have shown that ketosis is not necessarily harmful. In fact, the ketogenic diet, when applied correctly, is very safe and especially useful in obese or overweight people.

o **Does the green tea stop autophagy from occurring?**

Answer: the green tea's polyphenols induce the process of autophagy, they revitalize the overall health of the organism. The green tea is able to activate autophagy in the HL-60 xenografts by increasing the activity of the PI3 kinase and the BECLIN-1.

o **What does autophagy cure or heal?**

Answer: this cellular process is essential for maintaining a proper cell function; it helps to defend the cells in the body. It plays an important role in treating and preventing degenerative diseases and infections.

o **How much weight can I lose during the period of intermittent fasting?**

Answer: studies have shown that intermittent fasting that lasts from 3 to 6 months allows you to get rid of about 10 pounds.

o **Does the intermittent fasting put you in ketosis?**

Answer: according to the blood samples taken during some tests, the people who fasted for about 12 to 24 hours experienced an increase of about 60% in the energy produced from fat, with the most significant change occurring after 18 hours. This is the actual benefit of intermittent fasting, it puts the body in a state called ketosis. Be aware that fasting is not an essential condition for the ketones level to increase.

o **Is autophagy the same thing as intermittent fasting?**

Answer: No, but fasting can induce autophagy. In any case, keep in mind that the most important difference between intermittent fasting and autophagy is the purpose of the process. People usually fast in order to control their weight, while they attempt to trigger the process of autophagy in order to obtain protection against diseases and infections. Autophagy helps to protect the body system from diseases like dementia, cancer, and many others.

o **Does intermittent fasting detox the body?**

Answer: studies have shown that intermittent fasting has many health benefits, it lowers the risk of chronic diseases and infections and stimulate the process that helps the body to break down and recycle the worn out or damaged cells. So yes, it can help the body in the process of detoxification.

o **Does autophagy heal the liver?**

Answer: liver fibrosis is a common uncontrolled healing response to a chronic liver's injury caused by different factors; this is the end stage of liver cirrhosis and is responsible for a high mortality rate. The process of autophagy plays a vital role in the regulation of the liver's homeostasis, especially when it is under pathological conditions. It can help prevent pathologies like fibrosis.

o **Does autophagy reverse aging?**

Answer: autophagy funnels the damaged or worn-out cellular components into the lysosomes, where they are degraded and can be re-used as alternative building blocks for the protein synthesis and the cellular repair. The capability of autophagy to occur declines with age and may be less effective. In any case, its activation slows down the aging process.

o **Is too much intermittent fasting bad?**

Answer: fasting for a very long period of time is very bad for the body. The body needs vitamins, minerals, and other vital nutrients in order to stay healthy. Fasting for too long can be life-threatening, especially for people who suffer from different kinds of pathologies. Intermittent fasting, on the other hand, it's pretty safe, since you don't eat for just a short period of time.

happens to you when you don't eat for about 36 hours?

Answer: the body uses the stored glucose as energy and continues to function until you will eat again. After about 8 hours without food, the body will start using the stored fats for energy; for fasts longer than 24 hours, the body may start converting the stored proteins into energy.

When I finally do eat after a long period of fasting or nutritional starvation, will the food turn into fat?

Answer: at any moment you decide to break the fast, the body will be looking to replenish the stored glycogen in the liver and in the muscles at first. The body stores an approximate amount of 2000 calories in the liver; this happens because it is the easiest and fastest source of energy for the body to access and make use of.

It is only when the glycogen stores are full that the body starts to send excess calories to the fat cells for storage.

CONCLUSION

Giving space to autophagy, when you do it with an open mind, means to be ready to experience a lot of benefits. Through this book, I gave you a detailed description of everything you need to know about autophagy, starting from how it works and ending with some tools that will allow you to navigate confidently, avoiding the potential side effects. You are now, not only open-minded, but also more aware and able to understand the truth that stands behind all the different myths, benefits, misconceptions, descriptions, and many other things associated with autophagy.

I like to call autophagy the 21st century's key to a super healthy living. It is the best detox process you can experience, ever.

It's correct to say that we still don't have a complete knowledge about the work of autophagy in humans (due to lack of practical studies). In any case, it seems already clear that autophagy should be seen as a good friend and not as an enemy...keep it close to you!

One specific important benefit that I connect to autophagy's activity, is its ability to enhance cell resistance against environmental stressors. Our day to day environment has become more hostile in the last period of human history. Autophagy is here to tell you that you can make your body better, no matter what.

Autophagy amazes me, it's simply incredible.

Even with all the possible negative side effects, its positivity outweighs its negativity. Autophagy is good and healthy for you, this is the truth. I know this thanks to personal and direct experience. It's the best form of diet (and even detox process) that you can apply to your lifestyle. The benefits that you get from autophagy are beyond doubt much more advantageous than you can imagine.

Since I've started to enjoy the benefits of autophagy, I have experienced the excitement of a healthy life. That's why I feel obliged to share with you my knowledge, insights, and way of life. Employing and incorporating this into your life is your responsibility. You know what you want and how you want it. I'm sure that your life will have an incredible transformation.

I wish you good luck!

Yours,

Ashley Brain